A.D.D. AND SUCCESS

A.D.D.
and
SUCCESS

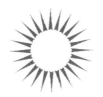

Lynn Weiss

TAYLOR PUBLISHING · DALLAS, TEXAS

Published by Taylor Publishing Company
1550 West Mockingbird Lane
Dallas, Texas 75235
www.taylorpub.com

Book design by Mark McGarry
Set in Goudy & Goudy Sans

Library of Congress Cataloging-in-Publication Data
Weiss, Lynn.
    A.D.D. and success / written by Lynn Weiss
        p. cm.
    ISBN 0-87833-994-9
        1. Attention-deficit disorder in adults—patients—Biography.
I. Title.
RC394.A85W442   1998
616.85'89—dc21   98–23898
                                                          CIP

Printed in the United States of America
10 9 8 7 6 5 4 3 2 1

Acknowledgments

A heartfelt thank you to the wonderful people who opened their lives and their hearts so that this book could happen. Your stories are available for others to learn from. Your legacy is already established as a result.

On a more concrete level, the actual writing benefited from my time-honored personal editor, Janis Dworkis, who helped keep my outlines concise and my words saying what I mean. Thank you, Janis.

Taylor Publishing Company personnel have again come through to construct a book of which I can be proud. Editors Holly McGuire and Camille Cline, Anita Edson and her publicity staff, Jim Green in sales, Lee Sommerfeld in special sales, and Carol Trammel, Art Director, plus all the others of my "publishing family" have my heartfelt gratitude.

Thanks to an old friend, Mike McLean, whose photo shoot produced the cover picture; you made "sitting" a fun experience yet one more time.

As a relatively new member of the Austin Writers' League, I want to acknowledge the support I gain from my hometown cadre of peers. This group of professional and novice writers have provided me with warmth, understanding, and tangible guidance and have taught me a lot.

And, finally, much appreciation to my agent, Mary Kelly Brice, who was instrumental in getting this project started.

Contents

Dedication

The writing of this book took on a life of its own. At first I thought of people's stories serving as models for those not as far along the path in their dealings with attention deficit disorder. It wasn't long after I started hearing the stories, though, that something else began to happen. Each individual's reaction to his or her life experience contributed to the change.

As the stories were told, the success each person had reached became magical, and I realized it was the magic of feelings that was bringing the book to life. The people being written about exposed their feelings, were willing to share them with you and me—feelings that give each of us the opportunity to learn and grow from others traveling by our sides.

None of us is alone on our journey. We only think we are when we're in hiding from the very feelings that can help us heal. Seeing them in another helps us face them in ourselves. Then we can recognize who we really are in all our wonderfulness.

All of the people profiled in this book have left an indelible impact on me as I lived with their stories, listened to their voices in my mind, and came to care deeply about them. Each brought a different perspective to the issue of ADD. Each presented a slightly different face to the way ADD looks. And each person has learned to live with their special, wonderful "brainwiring," solving daily problems in unique ways as well as constructing a designer life to live.

Perhaps it's the original way in which each person has become a success that has most influenced my memories of the person. If nothing else, let us all learn that there are endless ways to create outcomes, even when times are tough and our brainwiring doesn't fit well into the culture in which we live.

I have some sadness about the assault to the individuality of the people whose stories I've heard. But each has faced the hurt and anger and steered it into constructive use, taken feelings in tow and used them to advantage. That's part of what their success is all about.

One of the key reasons all these people made it into a book about successful people wired in an ADD way is because at some point in their lives, they decided not to buy in on the party line that there was something wrong with them. They refused to remain "cases." They threw aside the shackles of a disease/deficit model that would have left them in chains. And, freed at last to honor who and what they are, they decided to live life that way.

Over and over during the interviews I heard the same advice:

> *You must follow your dream.*
> *Live from the passion of your heart.*
> *Honor who you are.*
> *Find your fit.*
> *Envision yourself as fine just the way you are, ADD and all.*
> *You are a success because you're ADD.*
> and finally,
> *Find your talent, the passion of your heart, and know you cannot help but be successful.*

There's one more bit of magic, though, that needs to be shared. It took a little time for me to understand the impact of what I was hearing from the participants as they read the stories I'd written about them—comments like "It's a pleasure to see myself through someone else's eyes using my words" and "I blush every time I read this! Thank you."

One person said, "I really enjoyed it. It made me feel great." Another, "I felt overwhelmed. That was me in the story. Am I really like that? Awesome!" And another, "It was really hard realizing that I am a success, but I can't deny it now."

The magic has to do with the reframing of a feeling in every person I've ever met who is wired the ADD way, no matter how successful, skillful, or confident appearing. The feeling is one of inadequacy, of being somehow "less than" other people. So often I've heard, "If you really knew me, you'd realize what I'm *really* like."

In every person in this book, a transformation has either taken place or is well on its way. I didn't expect this outcome. Neither did the people I interviewed. But having their stories told truthfully, and in a positive light, challenged a long-held belief of inferiority. Just think what the world would be like if all of us could see ourselves through a positive filter. The besieged population of ADD people might just be able to break the siege and thrive after all.

I want to thank every person I interviewed. I gained much more than I gave. But their giving doesn't end with me. All of them know that many, many people of like minds, like hearts, and like souls will be the better for their having spoken openly and honestly. One has to admire the courage they demonstrated in being forthright about reliving their pain so that others need no longer feel alone, and I am thankful to have been part of this process.

These people have affirmed my belief that success has more to do with attitude, style of life, and purpose than with actual money, status, jobs, or relationships. These are all real people living ordinary lives. Each is respectful of others and cares about the environment and the future of our children. Each *feels* as well as thinks. And they are all doing the very best they can to live what they believe. What more can we ask?

I want to say to each of the participants in this book:

I'm glad you were born.
The world is a better place because of you.
Thank you for being you.

Yes, this book took on a life of its own. It's alive, filled with stories not just of the people who share their lives here but with your story, too. There's not a reader who cannot achieve the same success each person here has achieved. By owning and supporting a new belief in yourself—one in which you respect yourself and your ways as unique, acceptable, and just fine—you will create your own success story.

With each person taking that kind of self-responsibility, the world will indeed be a better place because of you. Please join me in being who you are. I also ask you to reach out to someone you may see stumbling and give a helping hand by sharing your own story. And when people don't grasp what you have to offer, simply ask them to consider broadening their perspective and wish them well.

In celebration, I dedicate this book to all who strive to live in their own uniqueness, honestly and with love.

LYNN WEISS

Introduction

Why I Wrote This Book

I was mad! Over the last several years I've found myself becoming increasingly mad about what I was hearing in professional circles about attention deficit disorder—ADD, the *disorder*; ADD, the *disease*; ADD, the *condition*. Even calling it a *difference* made my insides hurt, as if I'd been punched in the stomach.

The anger was actually a sign of progress on my journey of dealing with the whole ADD issue, with which I'd become intimately involved in the mid-1980s. For some time I had felt uncomfortable when I attended conferences or heard jokes about the way ADD people work or live. Even the self-directed humor that many ADD people adopt about the way our brains are constructed affected me negatively. Sometimes, the humor took the form of a passing comment from a spouse or parent that carried an embedded put-down—"Well, if you manage to stay married to someone who has ADD, you *are* a saint . . ." Often such remarks are accompanied by laughter and rolling eyes, expressing exasperation on the faces of people who believe themselves to be above reproach.

At other times I have seen people "telling on" themselves— "You *know*," said with emphasis, "who was the one late for the meeting." Finally, I became fed up with the whole issue of having to stand up and acknowledge, "I'm *handicapped*," in order to be allowed to reach a goal, do a job, or complete school work in a way that suits me.

My pain and agitation from these abuses has steadily grown over the years since I became involved with ADD. Even I perpetrated the abuse in the beginning, speaking the language of "handicap" and laughing at ADD humor over "our ways of doing things." But at last, in part thanks to my then teenage son, I began to listen to what was coming out of my mouth. He told me, "Mom, I'm *not* handicapped, and I shouldn't have to say I am."

I realized that I, too, was uttering the party line about ADD— one I was simply repeating without thought. I began to take note of the times when my stomach muscles twisted and my throat constricted in response to what I or someone else was saying about ADD. As a result, I realized that I was hearing subtle as well as blatant comments about the ADD way that make it appear something is *wrong* with us.

The issue came to a head when I was invited to be a co-presenter at a conference in which, unbeknownst to me, I'd been purposely set up in counterpoint to a medical professional who pathologizes ADD behaviors and ridicules ADD people. He places ADD in the same category as organic conditions such as seizure disorders and head trauma.

Here's what happened: In a small group of approximately thirty-five people, he introduced himself and spoke about his work with ADD. As I listened to his words, I began to feel tense and emotionally wounded. He likened people with an ADD style of brain construction to people who had suffered physiological trauma, who had *symptoms* and were *disordered*. They were, he said, in need of fixing. They needed to be "cured." He made jokes about his own family members who have a number of ADD attributes and generally talked in shame-producing ways about ADD.

As I sat listening, tension built within me. My head began to throb. I felt my throat constrict. And I felt as if a knife was being plunged into my midsection. By the time he'd finished, I felt as if I'd been beaten up and left for dead.

My turn came next. I could barely speak. I sat silently for some time, thinking about what I needed to say for those in the group and for myself. I recall pondering whether to put on my professional face and pretend I was fine. I knew I could do that, saying a lot of words, displaying my credentials, and basically speaking in a way I no longer believed. Or I could speak my truth.

I asked myself: Shall I display my humanness? Do I have the courage to say what is happening to me? Can I trust these people I don't know with my vulnerability?

I fantasized that I might lose all credibility if I spoke truthfully, but that argument fell silent when I thought about what I value in life. I wondered if I'd be further humiliated or perhaps confronted, if I spoke up. But decided I *had* to say what was happening—realizing that, ultimately, only I could deprecate myself. I resolved to respect the flood of feelings I was having and the probability that some other person might benefit by my speaking.

Finally, I spoke. I told how I was feeling. I did not put down the other professional, but I did declare the effect his words had had on me. I shared my pain. Then I followed with my perspective on ADD, a perspective that views ADD as a perfectly natural way of being constructed. Nothing is innately wrong with people wired in the ADD way, I told the group. And, in fact, the ADD way has value equal to any other mode of brain construction.

The result of my openness was—silence. The other speaker did not respond then or approach me in private later. No one in the group said anything. Only the next day did someone come up and say, "Prometheus lives." Not remembering the Greek mythology I'd once been taught, I didn't understand the meaning of the comment. So I asked. According to the story, Prometheus was the last honest man on earth.

A year and a half later, I still feel the impact of that verbal gift. At the time I wanted to cry in response to the comment. I felt like throwing my arms around the person who had said it. But, numb with emotional and physical pain, I simply said, "Thank you." I was drained. I had nothing more with which to respond.

Meanwhile, I nursed a migraine headache. Medication, which I rarely take, and sleep helped me to complete my duties at the conference. I stayed in the area for several days, enjoying the environment's great beauty. Rest and recuperation allowed my psyche to begin to make sense of what had happened. Slowly I realized how victimized I'd felt. Then, with renewed energy, I began to get angry.

It took time to harness the angry feelings so that I could begin to work with them. It took more time to detach from the individual who had sparked the feelings, to realize that he had only been speaking from his own perspective.

And it's taken time to implement what I know. We are only hurt by what we have to learn. Everyone is a teacher and this experience was a learning situation for me. That did not mean I had to remain a victim of such hurt. But I did realize it was pointing me in a direction I could take with my work.

To read the road signs, I needed to understand fully what I was feeling and thinking about ADD. I needed to decide what I wanted to do about my conclusions. In part this book is a response to those decisions.

For nearly a decade, I came to realize, I'd been given many clues that led me down a different path from mainstream thinking about ADD. For a long time, I now recalled and acknowledged, I had been uncomfortable with many of the words used in relation to ADD—*symptoms, over* reactivity, *hyperactivity, disorder.*

I also noticed that many of the so-called symptoms used to describe ADD were *interpretations* of behavior, with which I didn't agree. For example, the symptom called *poor organization,* typically attributed to people with ADD traits, is a gross generalization that doesn't really define that person's relationship to organization. Only in the last two years have I realized that many of us—for I have many ADD attributes too—who have a predominance of ADD attributes do have a fine, perfectly workable organizational system.

True, we often do not organize paperwork well. But when we use our innately strong creative and inventive abilities, we can be highly organized, if we are allowed to structure and time our work in ways that fit us. However, having spent years—even decades—being trained in ways that aren't right for us, we often have lost touch with our innate organizational capabilities. Even organizational details yield when we use an approach that fits us.

An example can be drawn from the way we approach a project. Rather than breaking a week-long project into five equal parts, we often do better accomplishing the project in one sitting toward the end of the week. The "all-nighter" follows several days of gestation. If you work this way, you might take Monday to learn what the parameters of the project are. You simply need to find out who you are doing the job for and what the goal of the project is as well as any other requirements. Then with this information tucked in the back of your mind, you can go about other activities during a gestation period. When you again attend to the job at hand, you pull out the guidelines and create the project all at once.

The completed project often turns out quite well. Organizing for it took place out of conscious sight in your creative mind. It was born whole. In contrast, others may prefer to place their organization plan on paper, breaking the task down into steps to be accomplished one at a time, day by day. Neither organizational form is better or worse. They are only different.

We're led to believe that intuition, creativity, ability to see the big picture, and the use of feelings are less valuable than systematic activity. Yet others who are constructed without many ADD attributes are not pressured to work in ways that don't fit. They are allowed to work from their strength, not their weaknesses. Ironically, they have just as many weaknesses as we do, only they have different ones.

However, untrained to feel good about how we naturally work, many of us who have a lot of ADD attributes have bought in on the party line that ignores our strengths and highlights our weaknesses, as if those are all there is to us.

On my journey to understand ADD, I vividly recall going through a stage in which I made up "diagnoses" such as IDD, Intuition Deficit Disorder, and GSD, Goal Surplus Disorder. Applying these labels to people who call us handicapped made me feel momentarily a little better. But ultimately I didn't feel good about myself playing the same game that I so hated when it was applied to me. I decided to find other ways to deal with the anger.

My anger boiled, culminating in a clear decision to *do something*. Rather than getting into an "us-them" oppositional mode, I decided to take a different approach. Telling people's stories emerged as one way to do this. It had the potential to carry a new message about ADD. It also carried the potential for diffusing my anger. Thus, I decided to write this book.

I also saw a desperate need for hope in those who feel bad about how they are constructed. I knew that support for being the way you are naturally brings pride as a replacement for shame. I knew that with new understanding, others can learn to weather the tough times. And with successful people as mentors, success is possible for everyone.

The stories that follow reflect my way of seeing ADD people using their ADD characteristics in constructive and wonderful ways. By knowing about people who have "made it," you and I can see the many ways in which people with ADD live successfully.

What is ADD?

When you can intuitively and sensitively assess how people feel, know what will happen next, or troubleshoot a problem, your ADD is working for you. If you can see the big picture quickly and envision how you might fit into it, you are experiencing your ADD skills operating. And when you learn by doing, get right into the middle of the action, or make up your own steps to do a job, you are also utilizing your ADD way.

ADD AND SUCCESS

Overall Perspective

The particular style of brain construction that is misnamed attention deficit disorder simply means that you deal with the world, in terms both of receiving, processing, and expressing information and events, primarily from a specific perspective— one not commonly valued in this society. Your right-brain, analog-processing, creative, experiential attributes all reflect the ADD natural way of doing things. In contrast, left-brain, digital-processing, systematic, strategic attributes all reflect a non-ADD way of accessing the world.

These two ways of functioning lie at opposite ends of a continuum. People in the middle of the continuum have 50 percent ADD attributes and 50 percent non-ADD attributes. There is no one place on the continuum that you do or don't *have* ADD. You merely have more or fewer ADD-style traits.

ADD is a *created disorder*. Although the brain construction is tangible and real, the labeling of this style as a disorder has been imposed by people who are constructed in a non-ADD way. Unfortunately, many of the people who conduct research or are scientifically trained professionals love to label and categorize and do not have many ADD traits. Sadly, they don't realize that their way isn't the only interpretation to be made from the evidence they view.

We also live in a culture in which most people have come to believe that the "linear" way is better. That's a judgment, again made by people who have few ADD traits. Even people with lots of ADD attributes have been trained to believe that they are less valuable or less *correct* than their linear counterparts. And it is this belief that creates most of the problems suffered by sensitive, intuitive, creative, big-picture people.

We live in a society where most people believe that there is only one standard, acceptable way to do things. It's considered the correct way. We live in a society that relegates differences to a category labeled "disordered" or "abnormal." I call this the pathologizing of ADD.

Specific Attributes

Rather than looking at ADD "symptoms" such as hyperactivity, oversensitivity, disorganization, impulsivity, moodiness, and reactivity, let's look in another way at people who are ADD. Those of us with ADD wiring:

- Attend to what is important to us, honoring what feels natural to us.
- Are just the right amount active to learn and work in ways that fit us in settings that fit.
- Have highly developed sensitivity that functions wonderfully well in many situations.
- Are internally organized in a different way than non-ADD people. (Time, for example, is defined by what's going on now, not by artificial segments called minutes or hours.)
- Concentrate without distractibility when processing information in our natural ways. (The school child can stay attentive when learning to make change in a play store that sells goods, but struggles with adding and subtracting problems on a piece of paper.)
- Are quick and spontaneous and move intuitively in many more contexts than do non-ADD people. We have a lower percentage of accidents than do non-ADD people.
- Have broad, expansive emotions rather than limited emotions.
- Seek and embrace feelings rather than control them.
- Intuitively know when to self-protect.

Forms of ADD

Depending upon one's personality, the outward appearance of ADD varies. It impacts the style of life we lead. Successful people in this book were chosen to show a variety of styles. For convenience I've categorized three types of ADD: Outwardly Expressed ADD, Inwardly Directed ADD, and Highly Structured ADD. Most people are a combination of two or three of these forms.

Outwardly Expressed ADD might be nicknamed the "Active Entertainer." If you have this personality style, you will tend to "act out" your feelings either verbally or through your actions. If you're mad, you'll probably mouth off, stomp out of the room, maybe even hit something. If you are happy, you more than likely will jump up and down or chatter like a magpie. As an outgoing person, you will be able to use your ADD attributes effectively in certain jobs, including sales and entertainment. You may gravitate to being self-employed or relish being called to solve a problem. You certainly won't shirk if a risk is involved.

Inwardly Directed ADD shows itself in the "Restless Dreamer." This personality keeps feelings down, tucking them inside rather than expressing them outwardly. If you have this side to your personality, you will be quiet at times. You are not likely to attract attention to yourself. When you get angry, few people will know it. If you're happy, the twinkle in your eye or a shy grin may be the only giveaway to how you feel. Jobs that make good use of this form of ADD include working in the arts, in crafts, and in building, fixing, and inventing things. You may be drawn to working with plants or animals or in the outdoors. Don't be surprised if you like to help people and become a counselor, teacher, or caregiver.

Highly Structured personalities make up the third form of ADD. I also call these people the "Conscientious Controllers." If you have a lot of this form of ADD, you will want additional control in situations that are stressful. If you become angry, you'll automatically try to control the source of your anger. You operate well within a specific structure but have great difficulty self-structuring. I first discovered this style of ADD in people who were successful in the military but whose lives fell apart upon discharge. Characteristic jobs that work well for Highly Structured ADD people include careers as pilots, in the military and in accounting, with computers, and doing research.

Few "purebred" types of ADD exist. Most of us are a combination of two or three types. For a predominantly ADD person to achieve a higher degree readily, Highly Structured ADD must be present. Many professionals have a little or a lot of this form of ADD. But the subspecialty in which you work will be shaped by another type of ADD. For example, an emergency room physician will be a mixture of Highly Structured ADD and the high risk-taking Outwardly Expressed ADD that thrives on excitement. A pastoral counselor would have a lot of Inwardly Directed ADD, whereas a preacher would be predominantly an Active Entertainer.

The stories in this book clearly reflect different personality styles. Each person has learned to work with the way in which his or her ADD style of brainwiring interacts with personality. As a result you will probably see parts of yourself in many of the stories.

Ultimate Perspective on ADD

It is my hope that you learn about ADD through the people in *ADD and Success*—people you will come to know as they share their lives with you. You will see how their successes are dependent upon their ADD wiring. You will be privy to what they've done to overcome the difficulties created by being ADD in a predominantly non-ADD culture. And you will realize that all of them have positive and negative attributes that help and hinder their lives.

The time has come to respect and honor the ADD way as valuable, just as the people in this book are valued as constructive members of society. Ultimately, I look for a world in which all people's ways are honored. I seek a time when ADD assets are noted with emphasis placed on strengthening them. I hope that attention is placed on people finding their *fit*—a fit that reflects how each person is naturally constructed. And finally, I implore all people to cease making judgments about differences and instead to recognize the worth of each person.

I envision all of us working cooperatively together, combining our talents. Visionary dreamers must work with detail-minded folks if a job is to be completed. Teamwork, not competition, must be the goal. Cooperation, not winning and losing, must be the end result of all our activities. Working together judgment-free makes this possible.

Choices Made in This Book

Intuition was the guiding principle initially used in my selection of the first people I interviewed. I also knew the individuals concerned, and I liked what their stories represented. Each had a message from which others could benefit.

Each person interviewed is successful at the time of their interview. No one can commit beyond the present. Their lives will go on for better or worse, but I also know they'll give their best to dealing with whatever they face. I can't and couldn't ask for more.

I understand that by my definition of success, no one is a hero; nor does anyone stay bigger than life indefinitely. Each of us has ups and downs. One day we may feel great, as if we can conquer the world. Another time we are sure that we are "has beens" or worthless. The successful people in this book are no different.

Initially, I asked potential participants if they would be willing to be interviewed so that I could tell their ADD stories. Some had previously been formally "diagnosed" as ADD, and others had not. In one interview I didn't use the words *attention deficit disorder*. Rather I talked about ADD characteristics.

I tape-recorded each interview, then typed the recorded material so that I would have verbatim remarks to include in the stories. Then I wrote.

Each participant reviewed his or her chapter and made corrections. I wanted to be very, very sure that all those interviewed were comfortable with how I had presented them; yet at the same time we all needed to be certain that the material was an honest and accurate portrayal of their experience. To my surprise, few changes were requested, and those made did not change the story line enough to make any appreciable difference in the content.

What you will read is how these people really are. I didn't "clean up" their stories to make them look good. I did concentrate on seeking out the wonderful ways in which each survived and is "making it" in life, honestly and responsibly. After all, isn't that what success is?

By no means are the people chosen for this book exceptional. I've made no exhaustive search to find "the best" or "the most" of anything that is supposed to represent successful people. To be sure, I have a token millionaire and a token physician. But these people are simply human beings, one of whom happens to make a lot of money and one of whom managed to get through medical school and find a branch of medicine he likes. And they would be the first to set you straight about their status in life.

Some of those interviewed are professionals, some are not. I tried to keep track of males and females for a fairly even split. But otherwise these are just people who were willing to have their stories told and who happened to be around when I was looking for someone to write about.

What Is Success?

The definition for success that I use here is different from the one with which I was raised. Then it meant money in the bank, a high-status job, and being the recipient of awards. The feeling of success was dependent upon approval from the outside world. Now I have another way of looking at success in life.

As with all of us, my own experience shaped how I previously looked at success. I listened to people "oohing" and "aahing" about what made up success, and I drew conclusions by watching movies and later television, reading newspapers, and going to banquets that lauded winners. As a result my early criteria for success were shaped by what others thought and said.

A decade ago I, too, had met many of my early standards for success. Yet something was wrong. I didn't *feel* like a success. It wasn't until I came to understand my ADD better that I was able to define the problem. When I did, I started a process of redefining success.

First I had to figure out who I am, *really*. I had to start feeling good about how I went about doing things. Then I had to begin to live the way I was always meant to live, authentically. From that I could feel successful about myself.

I had to find my natural ways of doing things and value those ways. I had to define successfulness in terms that fit me. I had to come to realize that my intuitive ability simply to *know* the makeup of another person was just as valuable as being able to be licensed to give a whole battery of tests to try to determine another person's psychological makeup. I had to affirm my desire to live the kind of life I want to live, rather than doing the sensible or safe thing. I had to make decisions based on feelings of my heart rather than on statistics.

In the process of defining success for myself, I came to realize that there can be no outside standard for success. Each one of us must decide if we have been successful doing what we love. We must ask whether we live the way our hearts tell us is the best way for us. We must ascertain if we've used our potential in constructive ways in settings that fit us.

My current definition of success does not rely on competitions, awards, or winners. It simply means that a person is living honestly, with purpose and kindness, being self-responsible and caring toward others. Success means being who you are at no one else's expense. And finally, it means learning from the past so that the present portrays a more whole, authentic, and in many cases "healed" person.

None of the successful people in this book are idealistic models of humanity because there is no such thing. I would not choose a wealthy person (even one who won awards for philanthropy) who judged others as worthy or unworthy. I would rather write about people who were at the bottom of the class but who hung in there, doing their best, than write about a straight A student who accomplished school work easily. And I'd much prefer selecting someone who has learned how to be a thoughtful spouse, even if married multiple times, rather than choosing someone who has stayed married to one person but rarely relates with any feeling or authenticity to that spouse.

As far as I know, no one in this book is currently an active chemical abuser or behavioral addict. None are engaged in criminal, abusive, or neglectful behavior. And none are such damaged human beings that they appear selfish, lack self-responsibility, or are hurtful to others.

The last major criterion for the people whose stories are told here is that each has an ADD style of brainwiring. And each has found ways to use ADD attributes constructively. Each has worked diligently to curb negative or troublesome ADD attributes.

We never fully change how we are in relation to our style of brainwiring—why would we want to?—any more than we can or want to change our skin color. But we can learn to accommodate and minimize the ADD traits that have not historically worked in our best interest. These people have done just that.

Successful people share their lives with you. I admire each. I thank all of them for their willingness to let others see their pain, their joy, and their realness. And I have received more from getting to know each than I ever was able to give. I know you, too, will experience rich rewards from getting to know these successful people.

Doug Meehan

My biggest frustration is with myself, thinking I'm not doing
  enough to get the job done.   DM

But, in reality, he is doing exactly what he needs to do to
  reach his dream.   LW

All during high school, Doug worked on a ferryboat transporting
passengers between Nantucket and Martha's Vineyard on Cape
Cod. "I ended up getting my captain's license," he says a touch
proudly, then adds with a slight hesitation, "that's another
story!" Smiling the captivating smile that makes him appear
about eight years old, he starts our interview by telling me a
story.

"You have to be licensed to become a captain. I had to go up
and take a test given by the Coast Guard. On one of the sections,
'Rules of the Road,' you had to get a ninety-five or better. It came
down to one summer when a bunch of us were getting ready to
take the test. The first one to pass could get the first mate's job—
kind of like an apprenticeship. You were no longer a crew
member."

Doug continues, "You had to have enough time on the water
to take the test. Because of my job in Florida that winter, I was
able to take the test early. It was a seven-section test. I went up

there, passed all of the sections and then got my score back on the section that needed a ninety-five. I got an eighty."

Watching him, I saw a look of pain cross Doug's face, followed by a laugh. "I'd have killed for an eighty in school." But he doesn't dodge that pain as he relates how he had to go back five times to pass that section of the test. The last time, "I didn't want to go back. Meanwhile, I was still a deck hand and one of the guys had gone on to be first mate," he says. "I didn't want to go back that fifth day. I asked myself, 'Why is it I cannot get this? Why can't I do this?'"

As a typically ADD person, Doug couldn't perform as well on a paper-and-pencil test as he could on the ferryboat. Clarifying, he says, "The way the questions were worded was very specific. They were set up to trick you, wanting you to figure out which answer from a set of multiple-choice questions was exactly like what was in the 'Rules of the Road' book.

"For example, a sample question might be, 'You are coming along during the night. You see a red light over a green light over a red light. What does that tell you?'

"Well, that tells you that there is a vessel that is restricted in its ability to maneuver. That's how it's worded in the 'Rules of the Road' book. They'd have that answer and then they have one such as, 'It's a vessel, due to some circumstances, that will be unable to get out of your way.' There were little variations between answers. No doubt could be present in your mind about what the answer was."

On a hunch, I ask, "If you were out on the water and saw that sequence of lights, would you automatically have chosen the right meaning?"

Doug's answer was clear and forceful. "Absolutely!"

In many ways, this testing situation exemplifies Doug's life. Bright, talented, and a hard worker, Doug feels, in retrospect, that this kind of experience helped him down the line in his present situation. "I got beat up so bad in school, mentally, knowing that when those tests were being given back I wasn't going to be getting a good grade, that I kind of got used to it. So today, if something doesn't work out, I say to myself, 'You can still have your dreams. You can still go for it.'"

Doug, a successful television news anchor in Austin, Texas, is doing what he loves to do—what he's wanted to do since he was a kid. As tough a business as television is, he has the life experience, stamina, attitude, and skills to keep on succeeding. "It's like a pyramid, this television business," he says.

Outlining a pyramid in the air, he points to the base saying, "Down here at the bottom there are so many people who want to be in TV. But," pointing higher up on his air-drawn pyramid, he continues, "as you start to climb up the ladder, up the pyramid where the great jobs are, people start to fall off because they say, 'It's too hard to get there. I don't want to do what it takes to get there.'"

But Doug is willing, and he's getting up there.

Doug's Background

Growing up on Cape Cod, the oldest of three children, Doug describes himself as having been a terror at home but a golden child outside the home. "I got into a lot of trouble at home," he says, "little stuff."

He spent his time out of doors, always playing sports in a neighborhood filled with kids who also liked to play outside. Football was his favorite game around home; baseball was his favorite in high school. He liked the social camaraderie of a team.

"My family is a typical New England Irish-Catholic family. My mother's full Irish. My father's half Irish and half French Canadian. Mom is very strong, outspoken and forward. Around the house, she runs the show. Dad, in contrast, is quiet, but as we were growing up, he had the humor and the 'fun-ness.' He tried to keep everything light and maintained an attitude that 'everything will be all right.'

"While we were young, my mom was a nurse for the Kennedy family. Then she went back to school when my sister, who's a year younger than me, was in college. Mom got a master's degree in medical ethics.

"Dad currently teaches library media studies in the middle school, in sixth, seventh, and eighth grades. He's now in his thirty-fifth year of teaching. When he started on Cape Cod, he taught fourth grade social studies.

"It was because of this job that he and my mom ended up on Cape Cod. They were both from Boston. In the summers, he would go down to my grandparents' summer home and after he and my mom met and married, he accepted a teaching opportunity and they settled there."

Growing up, things were difficult for Doug. But it's because of that difficulty that Doug is so adept at problem-solving and "keeping on keeping on." In contrast, his younger sister and brother had things come more easily to them, according to Doug. As a result, he feels his brother never learned to hang in there when the going gets rough. He's concerned about this, but aware that he can't do much about it—at least not now.

If Doug had to be described in only one word—as a child and as an adult—it would be "social." He's a good friend. "I have a solid core of friends and outside that circle I have other friends, who I just don't see that much because of time," he says.

Throughout his growing years, his natural proclivity was to "cut loose" and relax, but he was very much taught how to behave, and his father's and mother's influences clearly had an effect. Other than team sports—which he loved because of the social aspect—the rest of high school was "the pits," says Doug. "Awful!"

When I ask him why, the alert, obviously intelligent young man opposite me confides, "Because I never did very well in it."

The logical next question I ask is, "Did you try?"

Hearing the serious tone in his voice slightly takes me aback. Up until that moment, Doug had maintained a bright social facade—the one that has a genuine connection to his deeply optimistic nature. But in thinking about school, that facade gave way to grim feelings left over from nearly two decades earlier.

"I tried like the dickens. But I just . . ." Several moments pass before he continues. "It was very frustrating for me. What made it more frustrating was that my sister, a year younger, didn't have to try hard and did very well. So that's why when I graduated high school, I didn't want to go on to college. I thought it was going to be more of the same. And it stayed that way until I started visiting friends who had gone to college and realized, 'Oh, this is what it's like.'"

Doug took a year off after high school and went to work as a crew member on boats in Florida. During that year he applied to a college. "Someone said this college in Massachusetts had a great criminal justice program. I wanted to be a secret service agent. I had no idea where the school was. I had no idea what it was about. But I called my parents and said, 'I think I want to go to this college. I don't know where it is, but can you get me an application?' They did, I applied, I was accepted, and I sent in the check never having seen the school. I showed up in May and said, 'Mom, you want to ride out to see where I'm going to college in the fall?'"

So he planned to go to college without even knowing exactly where the campus was. I ask Doug how unusual this approach is.

"Not unusual at all," he replies. "I've done that a lot." For example, Doug tells how he moved from a job at a radio station in Cape Cod: he just got a feeling it was time to move on to the next job. And based solely on that feeling—because he didn't have another job waiting for him at that time—he turned in his resignation. A new job just kind of "showed up" right away.

But what if he hadn't gotten that new job? I ask. "I would have found something."

"Yep," I agree. "With your social inventiveness you would have found something."

Doug chimes in, adding, "And being willing to work seven days a week for three years straight helps." He's not kidding. That's radio when you're starting out. But I'm getting ahead of my story. Doug went to college to study criminal justice. He really thought that was the subject he was interested in. Was he ever in for a surprise!

"I started falling asleep in class and said to myself, 'Something's not right here.'" So one of my roommates said, 'I've got this Introduction to Communications class. Why don't you check it out?'" He did. And the rest, as they say, is history.

The irony, however, is that Doug had wanted to be in the television industry from the very beginning. It seems he was a big television watcher as a kid. "I'd fight with my sister because I would want to watch the news, and she'd want to watch *The Brady Bunch*. I always wanted to be on TV."

He'd asked his parents, "How do I get on TV?" But they had no idea. He continues, "There was no book to tell you how to get on TV. Only later did I find myself going back to what I'd always wanted to do."

Doug got into that introductory communications class and, not surprisingly, found that he no longer fell asleep in class. However, he did manage to get on academic probation every other semester. The core requirements caused him the most trouble. But his persistence paid off, and in five years of full-time study, he earned his degree.

The turning point came for Doug when a communications professor gave a class called Writing for Television. Doug found that he not only enjoyed it tremendously; he had a real talent for it.

"The writing was very tight, very concise—and pictures and sound also played a role in the stories," Doug says. "When I turned my paper in the guy slapped his hands together and said, 'We've found it. That's it!'"

It seems that when Doug had written papers and reports for the same professor previously; they weren't "pretty." Suddenly, they both realized that the problem was Doug's expressive skills. He could clearly express himself in the form used for television writing, but not in essay or report form. That's learning differences in operation!

Being the kinesthetic learner he is, Doug wisely started working for a radio station while in college. He says, "I wanted to do whatever I could just to get in. A buddy of mine down the hall was doing a radio show Friday evenings, seven to eight. I said, 'Can I go with you? Can I hang?'" Soon he took shift work at the station and began hands-on learning.

Radio and television is very much an interpersonal business— jobs are often found because you know someone who knows someone. And Doug knew that instinctively. "A year and half later another kid was working at a small mom and pop radio station. He was getting ready to graduate and told me they were looking for someone to fill in on Sunday nights, midnights and holidays—all the times no one wanted to work," Doug says. Doug's immediate response to being asked if he wanted to work was an unequivocal: "Yes, I do." Doug was on his way.

In 1989, he made a commitment to himself when he came to a crossroads. He'd been in a personal relationship for three and a half years and said to himself, "It's going to be one or the other, marriage or a career. I don't ever want to say to somebody else, 'We're married, and I know what I'm going for in my life, and I don't want to affect what you're doing. If you want to be with me, you're going to have to drop everything and get going.' At the time I didn't know where the road I was following would lead."

So Doug broke off the relationship and has stayed single. And he has climbed to his current job as a morning anchor on the biggest television station in Austin, Texas. He's in line to be "sold" as an anchor to an evening show but would actually prefer to become a game show host.

He likes entertainment better than news, and the current morning time slot offers him more opportunity to be spontaneous and to ad-lib. An entertainment-style show fits him better than hard news delivery. So, although he could play it safe with another anchor job, he's going for his gold.

Right now, he's doing a bit of "bungee jumping" by not securing something for himself in a few months. But he's hoping there is something out there that he can't see yet. He's willing to say, "Okay, I know what I want. It's not here yet. There is a safety net where I am. But I cannot do the safe path if it doesn't fit me."

When I First Met Doug

I first met Doug not because I was interviewing him for this book but because he was interviewing me—about a book I had recently written—for a segment on the local morning news. Leaving home at 5:30 A.M., I arrived at the Austin television station where Doug works in plenty of time for our interview. Unfortunately, though, it took a while to find someone to unlock the door for me. It was unseasonably cold for September in Texas, and there I stood ringing a bell that no one heard. Finally, I walked down an alley to the back of the building and knocked hard on a plate glass window—so hard that the weatherman, who was preparing to tell Austinites how cold it really was, detoured to let me in.

As a former radio talk show host and frequent television commentator, my body soon warmed as the pleasure of being in a studio once again got my blood flowing. I knew there were two morning news anchors and I wondered which one would be interviewing me.

It was Doug. And as soon as he introduced himself to me, I thought, "This guy is as ADD as they come." He not only passed what I call the "twinkle eye" test, but his walk, his talk, and his obvious sensitivity as he sized me up made him a likely ADD candidate. (I've never met anyone with a twinkle in the eye who's not wired in the ADD way.) We launched into a conversation instantly and didn't stop talking until after the on-camera interview. Time spent with him passed quickly, and I thoroughly enjoyed myself while observing that he'd done a good interview. He made me and my book look good. I appreciated that!

As I left the studio, I found myself thinking about him. I couldn't get Doug out of my mind. I called him the very next day, and he agreed to let me interview him for this book. We set a date for the following Thursday. I planned to go to the studio to tape the interview. Unfortunately, however, I didn't call him the day before to confirm our date. I thought about calling but then got distracted and didn't do it. The next morning I arrived at the studio and discovered that Doug had already left. He'd forgotten our interview.

Later that afternoon, he called me at home most apologetic. He told me how the appointment was written right there on his desk blotter, but he'd walked off without looking at it. He felt bad. I understood; after all, hadn't I, too, forgotten to remind him?

I don't worry much about those kinds of things. I've learned over the years to go with the flow, understanding that for one reason or another, I'll get a better interview later. Besides, half-teasing, I thought, "Now he owes me one, and I'll get a great interview because of it."

In reality we did have a great interview, and I've had the feeling from the moment I met Doug that he will be in my life for a long time. We've certainly not spent a lot of time together, but we hit it off like good old friends. He's got himself a supporter.

What Doug doesn't know is that I've got my eye on him as a

spokesperson for ADD and as a mentor and model for young people who fear that being ADD will rob them of their dreams.

How Doug Envisions the Future

Doug's future is what he dreams about every day. "I see my fifty-five-foot Bertram, a type of sport fishing boat, by the dock. I'll name it *Greased Lightning.* I've got my house already planned out with two floors, windows in the front, a nice living room and a great kitchen to cook in." He then draws the floor plan on the table with his finger.

"I love to cook, so then I'll just invite people over." With that you could see the twinkle of the social Doug radiating his happiness at providing an environment for the relationships he loves.

Smiling, he continues, "But this business makes me happy as well. I couldn't do anything else. In college, even though I'd never done any theater work, I auditioned for *Grease* and surprisingly won the lead role. I remember so vividly being in the makeup room. It was all a new experience for me. The show was sold out every night and I said to myself, 'This is unbelievable. What a rush!'"

Turning to me he continues, "You know what I do every morning now? I come in at five o'clock. I go in the bathroom, I put on my makeup and I go out there for two and a half hours performing every single day. And that's my rush. That's what it is!

"I want to encourage others to find out what makes their hearts race. Find out what gets a person exited to get up in the morning. And encourage them to go for it.

"I plan to keep up with a routine I began when I came to this studio," he says. "On my desk I have a quote on my calendar. Every month as I turn my calendar I rewrite a phrase on the calendar page. It says, 'If you can dream it, you can do it!' Walt Disney said that.

"I have to have a dream. Why not? And why not be a part of what the dream is. It's crazy to not have a dream."

I ask Doug whether he could live without living his dream. To emphasize further his awareness at only thirty-three, awareness that will shape his future, Doug emphatically says, "No. I was in a situation working for a high tech company right after I graduated from college in Boston. It was a start-up company dealing with phone systems for offices. I was going out of my mind. I said to myself, 'Doug what are you doing? What are you doing?' It was a wake-up call. I listened."

And by listening, Doug has created a life in which he can be happy. He is avoiding the awful depression and anxiety and frustration of doing things that don't fit. May he serve as a model for others as his future unfolds.

What Works For and Against Doug

One of Doug's greatest skills is his ability to read people. That's an ADD attribute. It's paid off for him in his career and in his personal life.

Thanks to Doug's sensitive, big-picture ADD view of situations, he's able to take what he sees and orchestrate it into a production. He blends all the elements before him into an expressive work for others to enjoy. Doug senses what people are feeling and is compassionate by nature. He pays attention to how he feels about situations and lives the golden rule, "Do unto others as you would have them do unto you."

He describes his sensitivity and ability to read people by saying, "I think, when reporting, how I come into all kinds of situations. Some are bad. Some good. I think how I have to be able to approach people in order to come home with my story, which is one of the reasons that I know ninety-nine and nine-tenths of the time I'm going to come back with my story.

"I'm not going to think, 'Oh, I'm not sure I can get this person to talk to me.' I know I can. My openness works for me. I don't believe in being fake or undermining somebody. I know how I am, and I know who I am and if I present that to the person, then I think I'm playing fairly. I think I'm a regular guy, so I think pretty much everybody else is just the same as me. I approach somebody the way I would like to be approached."

"What do you do when you are confronted with a situation where you're supposed to get a story, and it could hurt somebody?" I ask. His face becomes instantly serious in relation to the question, and then he smiles, saying, "That's why I want to be a game show host.

"I try to be as sympathetic as I can to a story and to a person. Everyone is a person, not a story—a person first. One Saturday morning, I was sent out to interview a father whose five-year-old daughter had been raped by a thirteen-year-old kid down the street. It's Saturday morning on a beautiful fall day. This guy is literally going through hell at home. And I don't even have a photographer.

"I'm the reporter and the photographer, so I have all the equipment and everything. I knock on this guy's door, and I'm going, 'There's got to be something else I can be doing here,' meaning, 'There must be something else I can do to make a living.'"

At that, Doug stops telling his story and laughs in an embarrassed way—a laugh that reflects the pain and understanding he felt about the situation he was describing. "This is not right. This is not right," he says.

"Not right by your value system?" I ask.

Emphatically, Doug repeated, "This is not right. I said to myself, 'Would I do this under normal circumstances? If this wasn't my job, would I go up to this guy and talk to him about his feelings in the situation?' Absolutely not. Let this guy have his privacy.

"There was nothing in the interview for the guy that I could see. I told him, 'Sir, I apologize for showing up on your doorstep on this fine Saturday morning. I understand what has happened to your daughter, and I am heartbroken over it. I have to let you know who I am and why I'm here.'"

"So you're strong enough to tell the truth?" I ask him. "It's the only way to go," he says, and then continues with his story. "I don't know why, but the man said, 'Okay, come on in.' I go bumping in with all my equipment and have to set up everything by myself. Set the camera up by myself, set the lights up by myself, sit him down, get his microphone on, go behind the camera, roll it and then run around and sit down and interview him. Finally, I had to get a picture of his daughter, a photograph."

I ask Doug how the interview worked out. "It felt good in the sense that I think I told the story that was there, the pain and anger the father was feeling. That's all I could do. I made a point—something that was constructive."

And he is equally clear about the point of his own story—the story of his life. Doug takes that clarity and becomes proactive in all that he does. It keeps him from being bored. "If I understand that I'm at the point of boredom, I do something to change it so I'm not," he says.

He also knows when it's time to move on. For example, when he was on Cape Cod in the job in which he'd learned and experienced everything he could at the radio station, he became aware it was time to move on. "I'd gotten to a point where I wasn't going to go up any more," he says. "I was going to start plateauing out. Once I recognized that, I said, 'Now is the time to go. Now is the time to move.' That meant jumping without knowing what was out there, but I knew I had to move on."

It was during this interview that I realized why the problem of boredom frightens so many ADD people. If you have reached your potential at a given moment but you don't act, you will tend to get bored where you are. For a lot of ADD people who have been taught to restrict their activity and deny their need for action, they become stuck—unable to make the moves that they might at one time have made naturally to reach their potential. This is the "good little girl/boy syndrome."

Even a tendency to be impulsive energizes a person to action. Doug's ability to be proactive also turns out to be a solution to the potential for problems with impulsivity. I ask Doug for a specific example of how his impulsivity shows up.

"When I decide I need a car, although I probably can't afford the car, I'm going to get it. My mind is set to get it. And I do it," he says.

"Then what do you do? How do you pay for it?" I ask.

"I do what I have to do to get it done. I don't leave a trail behind. I buy the car and take on an extra job to pay for it. I don't leave a trail of bad debt behind me.

Does Doug consider this a problem?

"No, I don't look at it as a problem," he declares. Then he hesitates for a time, laughs, and adds, "It could be a problem."

I wonder what is coming as he lapses into silence for several seconds, obviously thinking about how he feels and what he wants to say. I can feel the inner checking process that he uses to be sure he says how he really feels. He starts again by repeating, "No, I don't see it as a problem. I see that I know what I want, and I'll do what I have to do in order to get it, whether it means sleepless nights or getting up at three in the morning."

"So you always have a plan in your mind?"

"Absolutely."

In a way, Doug's unique relationship to his ADD-related impulsiveness reflects his proactive approach to life. It puts Doug in control of many aspects of his future. It feeds his confidence and inner security so that he can achieve his desires. He thinks before he acts, even as he responds to the desires of his heart. I believe we can all learn from this new perspective on impulsiveness.

Another talent that relates to Doug's ADD is his humor. He loves humor and can be very, very funny. A naturally talented, stand-up comedian, Doug feels humor is important in life.

He says, "I put on my yearbook that the best escape from life's problems is through laughter. I totally believe that still. I believe if there were more happy people in the world and more people willing to laugh at themselves, the world would be a better place for everyone."

As a friend, Doug comes out on top. He uses his ADD sensitivity and people skills advantageously. Nonjudgmental by nature—how can you judge others when you've been unfairly judged way too often yourself?—Doug opens his heart and soul to all people.

With a cadre of friends about him in his personal life, he experiences the peace that comes from being well nurtured. Because he is so outgoing on the job, he befriends those with whom he works, if they are open to friendship. There's no question in my mind that Doug uses his ADD positively in many areas of his life.

No doubt his ADD attributes make it possible for him to think quickly, improvise, and keep track of a million things at once while on the air. He's successful at television and radio because of his ADD traits. They work for him and his audience appreciates the results.

Though keeping track of finances is not a natural skill for Doug, he even has a way that works for this potential ADD liability. The creative bookkeeping of ADD people never fails to amaze me. When I ask, "Well, how do you keep track?" He says with a big sigh: "Not very well. Not very well."

"How's your check book?" I ask.

"Nonexistent."

My eyebrows rise at his answer.

"If I want to know how much money I have, I go to the ATM to see how much I have left. I look at the readout and say, 'Okay, that's how much I have left to play with.'" Then in a lighter tone, he says, "I usually have a running total in my head."

"You're not trying to 'beat the system' then," I say.

"No. It's the keeping track that I . . . I know that x number of dollars is going in the bank and that I'm spending so much on bills, but I'm not going to the checkbook every day." And so, using his creative ADD assets, Doug has eliminated the effect of any ADD liabilities.

WHAT DOUG WANTS YOU TO KNOW

Anything is possible.

Believe in yourself.

Believe in what you want to do.

If you can dream it, you can do it.

Milele Landrum

I find ways to get into trouble. ML

And she finds creative ways to get out of trouble. LW

Milele's rich, honeyed voice communicated a smile when she responded to my rattling off typical attributes associated with ADD, such as hyperactivity, organizational difficulties, impulsivity, moodiness, and temper.

Looking up from my note taking, I confirmed the humor I'd heard as she said, "Impulsivity? Well, I'd say I've got lots of that. I once pulled the chair out from behind my supervisor. Sure I was mad, real mad, but I didn't plan to do that. I didn't really want to hurt her. I just wanted to stop her. I was really lucky. Our boss gave me the chance to resign, and I took it, as quickly as I could."

Twenty-six years old at that time, Milele had not yet realized how many ADD attributes she had. Nevertheless, she knew it was in her best interest to accept that chance to resign. "The whole episode happened twenty-three years ago when my supervisor not only denied my request to leave work early but then turned her back as I was explaining my son was sick at day care," Milele says. "The child was only a year old and was having an asthma attack. I had to get his meds to him."

This episode was not Milele's first problem with impulsivity.

By her mid-twenties, those problems were already long-standing. She recalls that even in third grade, growing up in Paducah, Kentucky, she got into trouble because of her "big social-work heart," as she calls it.

"There was a guy who sat one row over and one seat behind me. He stuttered very badly. He was a really sweet guy and the butt of everybody's jokes. He had a very, very black, blue-black complexion, so he took a lot of heat. People teased him all the time about his looks, and he also had a very weak bladder. When he got scared, he wet his pants.

"Well, one day the teacher called upon him to spell 'Wednesday.' I looked back and saw the trickle begin to run down his leg. I stuck my foot out in the aisle and started to spell 'Wednesday' on the floor using my foot. Well, I was so focused on helping him that I didn't realize that the teacher saw his eyes were down and my feet were moving, and she knew I was probably doing something.

"So, of course, I got caught just as I was writing the 'd.' That's how I would stay in trouble . . . with things like that."

Since Milele "saw the ADD light,"—that's how she describes her response to identifying herself as ADD—she has begun to understand and be able to control her impulsivity and, for the first time in her life, truly believes she may be able to stay out of trouble. For six years now, she has been working successfully as a community resource specialist/trainer through a community college in Portland, Oregon.

Milele works with a welfare reform program and teen welfare recipients, assessing their academic needs, their learning differences—including ADD—the social barriers they face, and their entry-level career status. She receives high evaluations for her work and the promise of better things to come. She is a well trained professional who works hard to stay objective, while at the same time staying connected to her clients. "How can I not react to my clients emotionally? I feel with them."

Milele has made a breakthrough to success that she never thought possible.

Milele's Background

The oldest of eight children, Milele found herself in a difficult situation at age twenty.

"I was nearing the end of my first term as a college senior, expecting to graduate at the end of the summer, when my mother passed away." With characteristic humor, she says, "I was a senior in college on Friday afternoon and head of a household with five kids to raise on Sunday. My stepfather left right after my mama's funeral and got lost. The next time we heard from him again, he was dead. That was almost ten years later.

"As a biology major with little experience in life, I sure didn't have any real skills to raise my four brothers and sister. I didn't know anything about budgeting or disciplining. But I got all of those kids grown up and through school. We survived."

But it wasn't easy. And it took a while for Milele to understand fully the depth of her responsibility. "I remember a couple of months after mama died, I saw my little brother was running through the house and the sole of his tennis shoe was flapping. My thought was, 'They need to do something. The boy's shoe is torn.' Then it dawned on me ten minutes later: You are the 'they.'"

Milele's parents divorced when she was six. Her alcoholic dad was rarely around when she was growing up. He worked as a chef on a railroad during the week and had a second job on weekends. She now realizes that he was ADD, and that six of her seven siblings and her own son and daughter are ADD as well. One of her grandchildren has already been identified with ADD.

"All the women in my family have died young until it got to me," Milele says. At that point, it's my turn to chuckle and say, "You're too ornery."

In reply, Milele gives one of her wonderful gut-level, belly laughs and says, "I think I have a mission. I just didn't know what it was until I found out about ADD and how many lives it's touched and how much potential it has stolen from me, my family, and lots of people I know."

Milele's sister doesn't seem to have ADD attributes, though she, like their mother, is intensely focused—an attribute often found in families with ADD. Milele's sister has two advanced degrees, a home and family of which she is proud, and community involvement and the status that goes with it. She has made a place for herself that brings admiration from others.

The boys in the family have not fared so well. These are men whose lives have been destroyed by the ravages of unrecognized ADD: alcohol and drug abuse, the resulting prison stays, under-achievement, poor family life, and devastated self-esteem. Unable to succeed in the school system, unable to settle down outside of school, and feeling like the failures they appear to be on the outside, most of Milele's brothers have given up.

"My three youngest brothers are ADD, and none of them are doing anything about it," Milele says. "They are in and out of the criminal justice system for drug abuse. It's only when they use their drugs of choice that they can work and hold jobs and be semi-stable. But with the use of heroin when they can get it and crack cocaine otherwise, they end up in prison more than they are out.

"No one has ever understood what was going on with them. I didn't either for the longest time. They are high-strung. I remember when mama died, one of them would run away and break into the house of the people who bought her house. I thought his trouble was because our mama died. But looking back, that wasn't all of it. He never stayed still. He'd go with his dad, go with my brother, and stay with me. Later he had three wives at the same time. He was very impulsive, had a lot of jobs, and was in the army, navy and job corps. Yes, he's got a lot of ADD attributes."

Milele's family reflects the all too familiar story of ADD leaving a path of destruction through the generations. And this widespread destruction makes it the more amazing that Milele has "made it." But then no one ever said she was short on perseverance. It may not always have been pretty—and it certainly was never easy—but she's gotten the job done, over and over and over. And she plans to continue to do just that.

When and if any of her biological brothers, or spiritual brothers or sisters, ask her about ADD, Milele will tell them what she knows and assist them in getting the help that can make their lives different. But she won't push anyone who is not ready. Instead, she maintains her belief in the goodness of all people and prays hopefully that the brother or sister will awaken—perhaps tomorrow. Then they, too, can become successful in their own right.

Although there's no doubt that Milele continues to serve as a model for her family, she has had her own problems, too. Her progress toward the life she dreams of has been slowed by many jobs, her own drinking problems, and impulsivity and trouble focusing attention, not to mention an emotionally abusive marriage and a current partner with ADD. Her former husband was a womanizer and drinker who withheld emotional support from Milele and was overly critical.

Yet she's learned from every single experience and is putting her knowledge to work to help others. Now, she no longer needs to trade her self-worth just to have a man around, just to get attention and affection. She feels valuable and has self-respect, especially since she has realized the impact of her ADD.

Milele has faced her dragons, owned her addictions, worked her program, and pursued the question of why she is the way she is and what she can do about it. She points her finger at herself rather than blaming others. And she knows the difference between understanding why she is the way she is and using it as an excuse. That's why I consider Milele to be a successful ADD person. As we say in the recovery movement, "She's done her work and keeps on doing it."

It may have taken her 198 credit hours, several majors, six schools, and twelve years to get her bachelor's degree, but Milele did it—making As and Bs. And along the way, she learned how to work the system. Milele can pull standard English out of her drawer marked "educated" and speak authoritatively. Or she can slip into the vernacular of the street culture and, as she says, "cuss and jive with the best of them."

Milele's dual major of health science and social work has trained her to work with people much more effectively than with the mounds of paperwork that threaten to get her down. But throughout her work career—as a pharmaceutical and insurance woman, a social worker, and now as a community-college trainer—she has continuously developed creative ways to master that paperwork. She understands the difficulties faced by others who are ADD, and who are bright enough to do a good job if they have a little help structuring the parts of the job that seem difficult or impossible.

When I First Met Milele

I met Milele at an ADD conference in San Diego, California, in 1996. Her job had brought her to the conference. She felt she was missing something in her assessments of her students and thought she might learn something at the conference that would help her. As it turned out, not only did she find the help she needed for her students, but, as Milele puts it, she "discovered" herself. It was during this conference that Milele first recognized that she, too, was ADD. And her discovery has since been confirmed through a formal evaluation.

I first saw Milele while I was walking outside the conference center, surrounded by springtime's lavish display of flowers. My first image of her was of the sunlight reflecting off her sparkling white smile. In fact, she seemed to me to be all smile, emanating warmth of spirit.

I liked her instantly. Her wit amused me. It reflected a warm heart and a keen understanding of what was really going on. She "read" the conference and the presenters well. I remember thinking, "This woman gets it. She's got street smarts big time."

At the time, I didn't know what she did for a living. I didn't realize just how involved she was—or how involved she would become over the next year—in bringing forward an understanding of ADD issues in relation to welfare reform in general, and to teenage parents in particular. But I intuitively realized that she would both see the big picture and know how to implement specific goals that would actually help people—not pie-in-the-sky dreams, but real programs.

I also remember how impressed I had been that Milele had been able to pack up her things quickly and attend the conference when she received word only at the last minute that funding had come through for her. Rather than fussing about being inconvenienced, she focused on the positive fact that she was able to attend. And when there wasn't enough money to go around for conference housing, fees, and meals—Milele made do.

"So what?" she said when she had to take a bus across town to find affordable housing. "I'm here getting what I want."

We talked about her program and my current interests in training people in the skills that will make their lives better, despite being ADD in a non-ADD world. She understood exactly what I meant when I talked about people being cheated out of a good education because they were taught in ways that didn't fit them. She told me stories about the people she knew who were devastated because of unrecognized ADD. I understood when she talked about people not getting the services they needed to help them with their ADD—because they couldn't afford the expensive evaluations and medications that were currently in vogue.

We both knew we were on parallel paths to demystify and depathologize ADD.

But we also jointly recognized the pain and suffering that many ADD people experience. We agreed that what people believe about themselves is crucial to their success in life. If you think you're handicapped, then you are likely to act handicapped. If you think your way of being wired is just as good, but different from the next guy's, then you're likely to be willing to learn the skills to play in the world without discounting the wonderful way in which you are made.

Finally, I told her I was interested in working further with her after the conference. I often do this when I meet someone with whom I resonate. Sometimes we succeed, and sometimes our talking doesn't go any further. But Milele and I have definitely continued to develop our relationship.

A year after our initial meeting in San Diego, I came to find out just how much she'd taken to heart from what she learned at that conference. During that year, Milele integrated her learning into her program at work, developing simplified training material that fits her program's needs. A pilot program using the material Milele developed is in the works.

Not bad for one year!

How Milele Envisions the Future

Asking Milele how she envisions the future brings a change to her tone of voice. Seriousness replaces humor as she says, "To be able to get some real short-term modular training to the people who need it—training about ADD and how to live with it on a day-to-day basis. There are people I really care about who keep getting defeated because of ADD. I hope I have learned enough to help."

I instantly visualized several of her brothers, the special guy in her life, and some of the teen parents with whom she works. Milele's life is filled with wonderful people who are still chained by their particular style of brain processing. And I know she is particularly concerned about her young grandson.

"My eight-year-old grandchild has been diagnosed with ADD," says Milele, who has two children in their twenties. "I want to educate the teachers as he goes through school and educate my grandchildren as they go through life.

"The thing I look at now is this: Where would I be with the fire and energy I have, and the determination and love of knowledge and information that I have, if I had been able to control my behavior? My behavior is why I never . . . why in many jobs I had the responsibility but not the money or title of manager. When the position of coordinator of the present unit came open last year, everyone said to me, 'Aren't you going to apply?'

"But I knew I didn't want to apply because I knew I didn't want to go through that grueling process and be rejected. And I knew I'd be rejected—because I don't fit in those four-, six-, and eight-hour meetings with those suits. And somewhere in the process I'm going to call someone a—well, just use your imagination to fill in the blank.

"Now I'm content because I have other plans, plans that fit me better. I think there are thousands of teachers and social workers, probation officers and counselors, who deal with millions of undiagnosed, uninformed ADD clients on a daily basis. They know they could get to this person, but there is something blocking it. I know what it is. It's their lack of understanding of ADD.

"For people already employed, there's a lot of talent and ability that never gets touched. I know two ladies who currently work as administrative assistants but actually serve as the central nervous system to major employers. I'm sure both are ADD. They are just like me, only younger. Neither of them has the patience and discipline to get degrees. So they create and make do. Both employers would benefit greatly if these women weren't limited due to their so-called lack of education. I want to make a difference with all of these things."

When I ask Milele how far she could go in life now that she knows she's ADD and is getting some things under control, she says, "I think I can live comfortably, have money, not have to worry about the small stuff anymore, and be a major impact in the Pacific Northwest." Then, cautiously, she added, "If not even greater—though that part I can't verbalize yet."

"Why not?" I ask her.

"Because I guess that goes back to that old image and low self-esteem and all those other long-term demons you battle," she replies.

I laughed and say, "So you have a Pacific Northwest level of self-esteem right now."

Back comes the smile in her voice as her tone becomes musical again. "Yep," she says. "That stretches me. I think I can inspire. I don't know that there is a limit. Now, even as I speak, I know my biggest hindrance has been seeking out and finding the appropriate manager of my paperwork in order to bring all this together. I keep a lookout and know that it will come."

What Works For and Against Milele

Milele's success is shaped by the way in which her brain is wired and what she has done with that wiring. Some of her unique circuitry has worked for her, and some against her.

For example, Milele's ability to "read" people and work with them, one of her greatest strengths, comes from her wonderful intuitive ability to sense others—their feelings, capabilities, hopes and dreams. And that ability is clearly an ADD gift. She reads people's potential well. She also instinctively knows what they have to overcome in order to reach that potential.

By using this inner sense, she times her actions and teachings to match the readiness of the person with whom she is working. Without having to think about it, she knows when to put a hand on someone's shoulder affirming a move they are making, and when to give that Milele glower that can stop anyone dead in his or her tracks.

A person who shares Milele's ADD trait of sensitivity—the ability to read people—does not need to engage in lengthy testing procedures and diagnoses. The swagger in someone's walk, the "spacing out" during a conversation, the job-hopping history, and the "hyperfocusing" on one detail at a time—all those characteristics mean something to her. Not only can she determine whether a person has a few, a moderate number, or a lot of ADD traits, but she can tell what forms of ADD that person exhibits.

For Milele, these special skills are not just incidental. They are extremely important in her work situation, because testing and clinical interviews often intimidate and turn off the people with whom she works. Those procedures are costly and unaffordable by her low-income and welfare clients. Milele, in contrast, gets the same information "on the hoof." She's a true field researcher. And she knows it.

"My sensitivity," she says, "helps me the most because I feel what's going on around me and in my gut before it forms as a thought. I know."

Milele's knowing is bolstered by her awareness of the role she plays in a variety of situations. She's done a lot of work with her own emotions and behaviors and continues to work on herself. Milele has "walked the path" to overcome major pain in her childhood—the divorce of her parents, poverty, and racial bias. As she grew up, she's faced the impact of failing to live up to her potential and the problems created by broken relationships and addictive behavior with drugs, alcohol, and men. Now an active participant in twelve-step programs, religion, and her work with

ADD, she's found the guidance she needs to maintain self-awareness, healing, and growth.

Sadly, the naysayers who frown and glare with alarm, murmuring, "A complete evaluation is necessary to identify ADD"—meaning a clinical interview with a battery of psychological tests—often do not have the intuitive skills shared by people with Milele's sensitivity. They also are not tuned in to the realities of the world in which ordinary people live. Yet they may criticize use of the intuitive approach of identifying ADD.

In addition to her natural intuition, Milele's spontaneity and creative problem-solving—both special gifts of her ADD brain-wiring—also stand her in good stead in her work. Just as she "patched together" the skills needed to raise her five brothers and sister, she's patched together various jobs to make a living. Now she continues to patch together bits and pieces of money and programs to provide her clients with the training they need in order to be more effective in their own lives.

On the other hand, her spontaneity, positive outlook, and big-hearted nature—again, all wonderful ADD traits—have led her into some difficult situations and even worked against her at times, especially in conjunction with her impulsivity. She has spent hundreds of volunteer hours trying to help people, particularly women and children. And, occasionally, she has been hurt in the process.

"I would see their potential and act," she says, referring to the many people she has volunteered to help. "You can never tell if the time will pay off, and the person will reach the potential that you see. Sometimes you win and sometimes you lose." Looking back on these relationships, though, Milele says she now realizes she sometimes enabled people in a negative way, though never meaning to.

"One family—a mother and her father and four children—rented a house from me," she says, by way of example. "I had gone back to school and gotten this house very, very inexpensively. I decided to try to help this woman instead of look at other applicants. I even let her move in without paying the full month's rent.

"Months later, she still hadn't begun to pay me the full monthly rent, much less the back rent she owed me. Eventually, I had to have her evicted, and I felt abused and stupid. I had to sell the house to keep from losing it in foreclosure.

"I never did find out what the problem was. I wondered whether she had an active addition, saw me as a sucker—or what. But I know I did not help her or me in the process."

Was Milele hurt? Sure. Like anyone who lives expressively and fully, she has been hurt—but she doesn't linger on those times. Instead, she's made it her business to learn from what's happened, asking the question, "What's my role in what's happening?"

She hasn't always looked for, or understood, her responsibility in situations like this, however. But her involvement in a twelve-step program has given her lessons that she's taken to heart. She now sees a lot more clearly, recognizing when she's enabling someone else to stay dependent. She knows that spending her time helping someone else means she doesn't have to spend time working on herself. She realizes there's a balance between giving and receiving. And, perhaps most important of all, she's learning that she is a valuable human being worthy of being treated with respect.

Part of what works for Milele on her job comes from her sharing of her own "realness." Imagine how affirming it is for one of her clients to have Milele look her in the eye and say, "I am ADD and I'm doing OK. So can you!" Milele's not perfect, and she knows it. Yet she shares her story and her self, realizing that by telling her clients about her own ADD traits, she gives others hope.

Milele is making progress with her impulsivity, as she relates in this story. "I got a new boss along with a new assignment. I was real busy trying to get ready to move, so one day, when this boss gave me a flier about some training, I stuck it somewhere and that was the end of it.

"Well, we hadn't had time to get acquainted, so when she came on to me with a real authoritarian voice, just like my mama, right in front of everybody, I reacted, saying, 'Damn it! Get off my nipple!'"

Her progress at overcoming her impulsive tendency to blurt out emotional responses shows. Not only was she aware of what she'd done, but she stopped and thought about it.

"Well, there were students present as well as other staff. I understood what had to happen, because I know in a college setting that's not the way to go," Milele says, indicating that she does recognize what is politically acceptable in the workplace—even if it's difficult to get it right all the time. Milele both sees the big picture and is well on her way to learning how to set boundaries around her behavior to make her life more manageable. In turn, this will allow her to continue achieving so that she can work up to her potential more effectively.

"When I went to my first workshop on ADD, one of the first things I really started to look at was my ability to keep from saying the first things that come into my mind," Milele says. "I became a lot more conscious of my thoughts and impulses—saying things impulsively that you have to go back and apologize for later. I focus on a lot more self-talk. I talk to myself a lot now."

As a result, Milele had the wisdom to find her boss after that incident, so that they could have a talk. Because of Milele's awareness of her ADD, she was able to tell her boss what she needs so that they can both meet their goals of creating a successful program and a healthy work environment. After talking with Milele, her boss realizes Milele wants to do the best job she can. And now that Milele has taken the time to explain some ADD issues, her boss realizes she can make some simple changes that can greatly help their productivity as a team. For example, she can make a simple shift from telling Milele, "You haven't gotten that travel request to me. Get it done" to "I need your travel request by _____. Thanks for your help." And they will both be closer to meeting their goals.

Milele now knows how to educate co-workers and supervisors about what helps her be a better employee. This is an important skill that all people actually need to develop. But it is essential for Milele in order to overcome some traits that are not in her best interest to exercise. "I get saturated when I take a lot of information in. I have to let it roll around in me for a while. And then I use some of it all of the time, and some of it some of the time. Some of it I don't feel worthy enough to use—yet," she says. "But it's coming."

She succinctly states the goal of working with our ADD traits. "I'm learning to change how I think of myself. As I feel better about myself, I'm less sensitive in a hurtful way. I know when to protect myself and not try to do things that aren't good for me. That's all part of realizing how I am made—and that way is just fine."

I can hear her words now, "I am made just like I am, by a loving God, to add a unique flavor to this world." It is not surprising that Milele's name means "Something that will go on forever."

WHAT MILELE WANTS YOU TO KNOW

The reality is that I've always had this ADD, I always will have ADD, and there is freedom to live with ADD.

Consume all the experience and knowledge you can.

Use it when you're able.

Cesario Gomez

First you learn things by doing them; later you learn
to stop and say, "No." CG

And he's learned to think first and then act with
decisiveness. LW

As I observe Cesario, he chuckles softly with his deep-throated
expressiveness. He describes himself as having been much different when he was a young man.

"I learned what most young people have to learn," he says,
nodding and smiling softly. "Take, for example, where a young
person goes out and has a beer or something like that. That's
going without thinking. Anyone can go without thinking.
Maybe they try to do it again. Maybe all the thinking they are
doing is thinking about what they are going to do.

"There was time when I was like that—when I was in the
navy. For a while, I wasn't doing anything any good. The things I
was supposed to be doing, I wasn't getting done; so I quit
[drinking] cold turkey. I stopped. 'This isn't for me,' I said."

With an often repeated philosophical touch Cesario adds, "I
go my way even when the road goes that way." He nods his head
to one side as he says, "A lot of people go this way." Then he
nods his head in the opposite direction, "but I decided no, that's
not for me. It didn't work."

Then with his ever-present perspective about his Native American people, he adds, "A lot of my people try it [alcohol]. It doesn't work."

No, Cesario is not impulsive now, but he was when he was young—naturally impulsive. "Now I stop and think first. I learned," he says. Indeed he did.

To meet Cesario Gomez now, you would not guess that he had once been so different. This man knows himself. He is what he is and that's that. He takes responsibility for the way he is, and he doesn't try to be different. Neither does he judge his way of being as better or worse than anyone else's. Mellow, soft-spoken, and quiet, he moves easily in relation to his environment. He is a man of the earth, who works with horses, spending most of his time out of doors. In fact, he seems to be as much a part of the landscape as the animals and trees seen through the windows of his home and office at Taos Pueblo in northern New Mexico.

When I originally visited Cesario at the pueblo, I didn't think about the way in which his neurochemistry operates. It was unimportant to me whether he was ADD, non-ADD, or anything in between. But when I was considering who to include in this book, I thought of him again because he represented someone whose life was identified with the earth, someone whose traditional lifestyle honored a way of life that has been natural for many people for many generations.

Although Cesario is clearly ADD, I have never used that term in speaking with him. It somehow feels sacrilegious to me to talk about his, or anyone else's, naturalness in such "pathological" terms. (I aim to use the term less and less as time goes on, switching instead to a kinder, less judgmental way of speaking about this way of being constructed; but it's difficult to abandon the term in a book like this.)

What my relationship with Cesario has so clearly shown me is what I already knew to be true: when a person lives in a more natural way than most of us can, so close to the land, ADD tends to disappear as a disorder. Instead, the ADD way of being exists as the absolutely most appropriate, natural way of living. In Cesario's personal life and in his work, almost all of his ADD traits are simply the normal and best way of doing things—the only significant exception being his impulsivity when he was much younger.

And this makes me realize once again that the difficulties so often caused by ADD are not really difficulties at all. They are simply conflicts between this particular group of natural traits and the "digital" structure that is superimposed on those of us who live fast-paced lives, working in large institutions in large cities.

Consequently, instead of making an issue of the term ADD when I was with Cesario, I spoke about "Indian thinking"—all the while observing behaviors and listening to language that we usually identify with ADD.

Cesario, like all analog processors, tends to learn by doing things firsthand rather than by talking or reading about them. He "goes with the flow," is creative, sensitive and intuitive, often effectively using feelings as a guide. To Cesario, the journey tends to be more important than the goal. It's not that he doesn't have and reach goals—he has set and reached many goals; it's just that he reaches them in his own way, frequently creating an experience in the process.

Cesario's Background

A handsome man in his fifties, Cesario arrives for our meeting in his pickup truck wearing jeans, boots, and a cowboy hat—all of which strike me as natural in the Southwest as wearing a three-piece suit does in the city. We begin to talk about his life.

"I was born in Taos Pueblo, grew up in Taos Pueblo, went to school at the Taos Day School at the pueblo," Cesario says. He speaks emphatically at first, using curt phrases and often leaving out connective words, such as "and." He has a good vocabulary and excellent verbal skills, but he sometimes chooses not to fool around with a lot of fancy rhetoric. I suspect that his apparent reticence at the beginning of our interview stemmed from being mildly ill at ease—partly because he learned a long time ago not to trust someone who was "European," meaning non-Indian, and a woman to boot. But he is a gracious person, polite and generous with his time.

A true western gentleman, Cesario has a life to which I'm not privy—a part of his life he chose not to reveal during our conversations—and I respect that. Sandi, his wife, alluded to it by saying Cesario was just coming into his "elder years"—the time when adults begin to be considered wise. I do know that he is a respected mainstay of the Taos Pueblo community, an active member of the Tewa tribe, and a model for the youth. A dedicated family man, he guides and educates his own children and grandchildren in the ways of his people. And he cares about all the Indian children in the village as if they were his own—one big family.

The school Cesario attended as a child was run by the U.S. Bureau of Indian Affairs. When asked what it was like, he says, "It was kind of hard, because there were a lot of Indian kids who spoke the Tewa language. It was hard to really speak English well. All the lessons were in English."

Cesario attended that school through the seventh grade before deciding to go into town, because "I wanted to speak only English." He finished high school at Taos High, which he says he found interesting. Much of his time was spent in athletics. "I played it all—football, basketball, baseball, ran track. It was a lot of good stuff," he says, smiling at the memory of those early years. Then he continues, "I was a pretty good athlete, both quick and strong."

I can imagine Cesario lifting weights and throwing the javelin in track, running long distances and playing both offense and defense in football—playing the whole game. As he puts it, "I had the stamina to hold up."

Academically, Cesario liked learning new and different things every day. As with many students with ADD, that novelty was what held his attention. Math was his favorite; history was not, he says, partly because history meant reading. As he puts it, "Reading has never been real friendly for me. If something is very interesting I can follow it. If not, I put it away." To this day, he feels the same way.

"Something that is very interesting, like government or politics, I'll read about it. I read the paper every morning. When the paper does not have interesting copy, I get to thinking about other things, like having a lot of animals to take care of. So, I get up, and out I go to check on them. But if the material holds my attention, I don't think about the animals right away."

The second boy in a family of four boys, Cesario was raised "in a very nice family—kind people who are caring, family-minded and thoughtful." He describes his mom as "a pretty well-educated lady." Then he adds, "She died when I was seven years old." From that time, Cesario's father took care of him and his brothers. Another woman in the family also helped raise the boys, but it was "kind of hard."

Thoughtfully, Cesario adds, "It turned out to be rough. My dad was a very strong man, hard working. Only going to school as high as the third grade, he had to do what he had to do." That meant a variety of jobs including "working a dairy, a lot of cattle and a lot of trucking, moving stuff from Colorado to Taos. We boys learned how to drive tractors and stuff like that and to work the cattle." Cesario and his family know all about how to do a day's work.

Lowering his already soft voice, he continues to talk about his dad. "He was a wise man. A very wise man. In the Indian ways he was pretty highly educated. In teaching the younger people religious stuff, the traditions, he knew everything about them. He had a real good memory for the history, the stories and the rituals."

Each of the boys in the family acquired a trade. Cesario attended a government-run trade school after graduation from high school. "I went to Lawrence, Kansas, to learn to weld," he says. "I wanted to be an artist, but then decided I didn't want to come back to Taos any more."

Speaking about himself, but also for many young Native American people, he explains, "When you're from a Third World country, you want to have a life, so you want to go where there's life—where you think there's life." This urge for a different lifestyle led Cesario to California, where he was readily employed as a welder. "The money was good, and I was happy. Then Uncle Sam got me. Everything changed.

"Uncle Sam caught up with me. They were going to send me to the army. 'No way,' I said. No target practice for me. So I joined the navy so I could see the world. I went to Santa Fe to get in the navy, and they sent me to San Diego, California. I spent four or five years, mostly in the Philippines."

That was when he met a young white woman named Sandi, in California. She was waiting for him when he "came in from the ocean on a big ship." Smiling, he says, "There was this lady standing there withn her lariat, swinging it like this," at which point Cesario demonstrates his throwing technique with an invisible rope. "She was there. She got me right around the neck, so I got married.

"The lariat came first and then the hook, and here I am," he continues with a sly smile, "still married thirty years later." He chuckles at his own joke.

I wondered how and why Cesario and Sandi ended up back at

the pueblo? Cesario's answer came in story form, as he described his thinking one night while standing duty on the ship.

"I was standing there on the deck and the question occurred to me: 'What am I doing here fighting somebody's war, and my people are in the United States fighting the United States government, trying to fight to get back our land?' That's kind of what brought me back here—to do what I could do."

Unable to find work quickly upon his return, Cesario decided to go into business for himself. The desire to become an entrepreneur, and the ability to see creative solutions others might miss are ADD traits that have worked well for Cesario.

With Sandi's help—he generously attributes a lot of his success to his wife—they started a horse ranch that is now in its thirtieth year of uninterrupted operation, providing outdoor activities for both tourists and locals. Their clients find the Gomez ranch experience inviting, fun, and inspiring. And having participated in some of the activities myself, I can attest to the memorable nature of time spent at the ranch.

So I wasn't at all surprised to hear Cesario say, "People tell me how I make their vacation. I put them on a horse and take them out, and they have a wonderful time." The business that has supported Sandi and Cesario and their four children reflects their joint efforts. Sandi does the office paperwork, acting as the organizer, scheduler, and planner. Her skills are well suited to these tasks, which are often difficult and sometimes frustrating for people with ADD. Equipped with the gift of gab and acting as receptionist, Sandi is often the first person at the ranch with whom potential clients have contact. In contrast to Cesario's softly spoken, short phrases, Sandi provides a lively travelogue and review of the wonders awaiting you at the horse ranch.

Cesario is in charge of the "outside world," the horses, riding lessons, the acreage, and other activities such as rafting.

"I like horses. They're big and gentle," Cesario says. And he adds with humor, "One important thing about horses. You train them, you feed them, water them, take good care of them, and you can yell at them and they don't talk back at you. That's what I like about them." But to watch Cesario with his horses, you recognize instantly the incredible respect he has for each four-legged animal in his charge. The special intuition that allows him to communicate so well with these animals is another ADD trait that has been a gift in his life.

Cesario and Sandi also put out a small newspaper four times a year. Sandi does the typing, some of the writing, and the layout. Cesario goes over the layout, too, and sees to advertising and distribution. The newspaper advertises local businesses, provides a guide to local activities for tourists, and serves as a source of historical information and political articles. Subject matter covers the history of northern New Mexico and the pueblo, craft techniques, and spiritual guidance, as well as pending activities and parenting and self-help information for healthy, balanced living.

As you can see from this example, Cesario and Sandi perfectly embody the concept of "teaming," in which two people's different strengths are added together to create a whole. Each one's weaknesses are compensated for well by the other person. As a result each accomplishes much more when they tackle life together than they could individually.

It's been a full life so far for Cesario. He has seen his children grow and he has nine grandchildren, a successful business, and respect from other members of his tribe as well as from the community.

When I First Met Cesario

I first met Cesario and Sandy some ten years ago, when I was in Taos for some "R and R." I found myself flipping through several pamphlets in a local motel room. Suddenly I spotted a photo of horses and thought, "What a great way to see some of the local geography while engaging in a favorite activity, horseback riding!"

Sandi's chipper voice greeted my inquiries and answered my questions, so that I soon found myself standing near the horse ranch corral. It felt good. I noticed a husky, stately looking man who seemed to be in charge of the ranch. He was saddling horses and talking to them. Of course, he was Cesario.

As the evening colors began to overtake the bright afternoon light, he led me and two other people on a dusk ride over sandy land covered with sagebrush. I had a wonderful time and was treated to a considerable amount of history, cultural lore, and explanation of what I was seeing. I knew at that moment that Cesario was definitely a reflection of the environment. Later, I learned that he is a full-blood Tewa Indian whose Indian name is Stormstar. Back at the office I found out that Sandi also has an Indian name, Willowwoman.

As I was getting ready to leave, a writer appeared to do a story for a major national newspaper. He was there to interview Cesario and Sandi about a program designed to rehabilitate Indian kids who were having trouble with alcohol and other chemicals. By participating in traditional activities, horse riding, camping, swimming, and pack trips at the pueblo, and by being exposed to the true history and lore of the Tewa, many of the kids were changing for the better. Learning about and taking pride in their history meant they could begin to take pride in themselves and their behavior. The program was working. And the newspaper wanted to tell the story.

Cesario and Sandi obviously cared a lot about these kids and were willing to work to turn the tide of chemical-dependency problems around. To this day, they continue to work with youth, now often from inner cities, who need to find their spirit in an environment where one can think rather than simply react.

How Cesario Envisions the Future

Cesario envisions his future by following the desires of his heart as he sees the needs of his people. As already indicated, his natural intuition, sensitivity toward other people and animals, and rich emotional life are all ADD traits that have been positive forces in moving him toward his goals and toward the dream of helping his people.

Cesario is already living his future through the manner in which he approaches life. He is "walking his talk." Not only does his life serve as an inspiration, but when he shares his story with others, he uses the time-honored approach of storytelling to teach and empower. Young people, as well as other adults, can be guided by Cesario to think through their own stories, choose what to believe in, and live for the greater good. Many of Cesario's goals for the future involve the tribe: getting money for the tribe, buying back the land, rehabilitating the youth, and righting the wrongs taught historically.

Now he tells Indian kids, "If you don't speak up, it reinforces the government's belief that the only good Indian is a dead Indian." He says, "I talk to them and tell them to get off the drugs and alcohol. I tell them the way it really is.

"When I'm talking to a European kid, I say, 'It's just one less European if you don't get this right.' I sit the kid down and talk to him about life just like I'd talk to an Indian kid. I'd ask if he wanted to be a drunk or a drug addict or does he want to live life the way other people who are successful live. I ask, 'Do you want to be a failure? Why are you hiding?'

"I ask all kids, 'If you're looking for a doorway out, then I'll help you.' I explain about the facts of life. Most important I tell the kid, 'If you're young and alcoholic or a drug addict, you can't help anybody.' I pray for that person and try to help him go the right path.

"I spent a lot of time with a kid here in Taos, helping him along. He'd do pretty good for a while and then he'd fall. Then he jumped to the next city and to the next city and to the next. I tried to tell him the direction he was supposed to be going, but he wouldn't listen."

Wondering why Cesario thought a child might act like this, I ask, "What gets in the way of such a youth being able to listen?" And he answers with wisdom born from his natural intuition and sensitivity.

"Being abused since he was small. He doesn't trust. That's the problem. Some kids don't trust—usually because of abuse. Some are confused. Some can't let go of the past, and they go back and do something they shouldn't be doing. They use drugs. They run. They don't stop and fight it [the feelings], because they have it [mistrust] in there [inside their gut] since the time they were small."

He continues, "There are some who will fight what I call the demon. They will fight it, and they will go on beyond it and leave that behind. Those are the ones who will make it."

Once quiet, Cesario speaks up these days and, with Sandi's help, writes about the plight of the Taos Indians and Indians in general.

"I learned to keep quiet in school," he says. "You see that when you grow up and have learned American English so you can read, you find out that all the stuff taught in school as a Native American doesn't make sense. So it's kind of like, 'Why am I doing this?' I mean stuff like finding out how the Spanish and Christianity and the U.S. government treated Indians so badly from way back.

"The people at school were trying to teach us this stuff, trying to make us understand. But what is there to understand about? I remember thinking, 'You killed our ancestors, sixty million Indians.' What's to understand?"

As a youngster Cesario kept quiet about what he was expected to learn that didn't make sense to him. But no more! Now he teaches history the way it happened. He speaks up and plans to continue to be a force in his village. Not one naturally inclined to public speaking, he plans to continue working quietly—but no doubt effectively—for the rights of Native Americans.

What Works For and Against Cesario

As discussed earlier, Cesario's ADD traits create few problems for him because of the lifestyle he has chosen to live. In fact, most of his ADD traits have been positive forces in his life.

One difficulty Cesario has had, and a common one for many people with ADD attributes, comes when he is required to put things down on paper. This is simply not something that comes naturally to him. And he avoids it whenever he can, often by trading tasks with Sandi.

But unlike many people, who are required to put their ideas on paper or think they need to, Cesario doesn't really need to put things on paper. That's because he can visualize problems, images, and solutions so easily in his mind's eye. How does he do it?

"When I'm building something, I would have a hard time if I put it on paper first," Cesario says.

"So you go right to building it?" I ask.

In his precise way, he corrects me: "Actually, I put it in my mind first, then apply it. I learned to do that. I study it. Whatever I want to make or build, I study it. I just turn it in my mind like a window frame. Then I build it. If it doesn't turn out right, I go back in my mind, and change things. First I do it in my mind, and then change it however it needs to be changed. I can take what's in my mind and have it come out of my hand."

Cesario also uses his internal visualization skills to sketch memory pictures of the old people who passed away a long time ago when he was young. "I sketch them exactly the way they looked, which I kept in my mind, and it comes out the way I see it."

Cesario is aware of his intuitive—almost psychic—skills. And he told me the following story that illustrates their use.

"One time we went on a river raft and took my whole crew—about fourteen. I was just lying down on the raft. We were going downstream and everybody was happy. All of a sudden, it was like something had happened. But I looked around and the water was real smooth, real smooth. The feeling didn't make sense, but I kept looking around feeling like something would happen. I didn't know what it would be. I felt it."

Having built expectations within me wondering, knowing, for sure that something was going to happen, I waited for the rest of the story. And it came.

"We turned around the bend and saw the bridge. And right away I knew something would happen. Some people were throwing boulders into the water from that bridge. When the boulders hit, the water would go twenty feet up in the air. The boulders could have killed someone." Obviously, Cesario and the others made it out okay, thanks to Cesario's words of caution.

I ask Cesario if he considers this intuition to be a part of Indian thinking.

He answers, "It's just kind of a sense that something is going to happen, and you don't know what it is, and you are fighting in your mind, 'What is it? What is it?' Then it happens and then you know."

And at that, he laughs the laugh of self-awareness and acceptance brought about by living through many experiences. Now Cesario accepts such feelings as natural.

I suspect Cesario reads people well, too—their motives and intentions—so I ask if his intuition works for him in relation to people.

45

"You talk with people and soon you understand where they are coming from," he answers. "If a man is a lawyer or a doctor or a construction worker—by talking to them, the way they sound, you try to figure out what kind of person it is. I sense what they are about. And I just know when the person is not being real. I feel it in my gut."

"Are you usually right?" I ask.

"Just about every time—on target," he says with a twinkle in his eye and some delight in his voice.

Another trait that works in Cesario's favor is his anger. Not only is anger an understandable emotion considering the history of his people, but Cesario seems to be using his anger constructively to right some wrongs.

"I sit and watch. I see what the government is doing to this country and what they are doing to each other—how they [Europeans] are destroying themselves," he says, in discussing his anger. Then he turns to me and asks, "Do you know there are a lot of non-Indians coming to the New Mexico area?"

I nod and prompt, "And . . .?"

"They are grabbing things. It's always, 'Give me this or give me that, so I can get some money.' For example let's say I create a beautiful sculpture, and you want it, and you give me money for it. Then you turn around and sell it for more. That's what I'm talking about.

"Now that we have a little something created—gambling—tourists are coming here and some of the money is staying." Then he adds, "I don't like gambling, but I'm for it."

He uses an analogy to explain what he means. "If I'm fighting you with a bow and arrow and you have a cannon, now I like the cannon. With gambling I'm fighting the government. That's the only reason I like the gambling. With money we have a chance to fight the state.

"Now, we can go up the ladder potentially. When it comes to

money, if you have money, you can fight for our land. We lost so much. We lost some self-governing power in 1996. Now we're trying to buy back some of our land right here on the mountain, helping the children, watching out for the Indians and all kinds of things like that. So, what this whole thing boils down to is how we're fighting to stay alive." Cesario uses his anger, which is considerable, to work through "channels" to help his people.

Cesario's story—and the story of his people—is not dissimilar to the story of ADD people who have been stripped of their power to learn, work, and express themselves freely using their innate ADD wiring. The intuitively skillful teacher who must pass linear licensing tests in order to teach, or the talented engineer who can fix anything but can't get a diploma to prove it, are only two of many examples of the kinds of stumbling blocks faced by many people with ADD wiring.

Perhaps Cesario is onto something from which we all can learn. There does seem to be a time for righteous anger, used "within channels" to right wrongs that one sees. This may be the time to honor truly the idea of diversity by providing diverse ways that people can demonstrate what they know and how they work. Let us work together.

Cesario has also managed to overcome the effects of some of the potential handicaps of ADD. By choosing as a companion someone who has the skills to organize paperwork and keep up with it, and who is willing to work with him, he has overcome the problem of providing a skill with which he is not naturally endowed. I wonder what Cesario thinks would happen to him if someone tried to keep him behind a desk.

"It wouldn't work. I don't have the patience to be sitting there." His humor quickly surfaces again as he adds, "I don't think my rear end would hold out. I am too heavy to be sitting at a desk all day long. I would get some blisters. Some people can sit that way, but me, I would feel like I was getting old just sitting there. I gotta be out there doing something, something that I can see that it's kind of growing, or train a horse, or teach a person or help somebody. That's me!"

Cesario is a man who knows himself. He takes responsibility for being that way and doesn't try to be different. He is what he is.

WHAT CESARIO WANTS YOU TO KNOW

Stay in school.

Stay off alcohol and drugs.

Walk your talk.

G.B. Khalsa

If I were to list all the things I do, you would be
mortified. GBK

Yet she does them gracefully and well. LW

Sitting outside G.B.'s quilting shop in Wimberly, Texas, on a
porch made of fieldstone, I discover once again how fortunate I
am to be able to interview people for this book. A slight breeze
stirs the hot September air; a few late-blooming wildflowers wave
at us and the plantings throughout the craft complex provide an
atmosphere conducive to leisurely conversation.

As I'm in the process of settling in—I test my tape recorder
and adjust my chair on the uneven floor while G.B. arranges the
handwork she's brought to keep her busy while we talk—G.B.
quietly pops out of her chair. (She moves so silently and effort-
lessly that you don't realize she's going anywhere if you're not
looking at her.) She ducks around the corner and drags out a
quilting frame with her current project stretched across it.

She laughs gently, two projects within easy reach, and says, "I
focus better when I have something in my hands." We both
laugh, knowing the truth she has voiced about people like us—
creative, active ADD people, who do indeed listen and sit still a
whole lot better when we have something to do.

49

Midwife and quilter, G.B. prefers a life that is filled with variety.

"I started wanting to do something similar to my quilting shop fifteen years ago. I was a midwife then and felt that I needed something for balance to recharge me," she says. "I consider the act of birthing so holy that you get a lot from it, but it has quite a bit of stress, especially in modern society.

"To be a midwife is very romantic to people. But, in reality, it's not accepted," she continues. "Listen to the average American family's conversation when their daughter tells them she's going to have her baby at home. It's not unusual for the parents and grandparents to 'freak out' and even sometimes offer to pay the hospital bills.

"We also get hassled a lot by the medical community with abject, unbelievable rudeness. It goes on and on and on. So what I usually do at a birth when I need to calm myself and become focused and mindful and non-intrusive is handwork."

G.B. speaks lyrically, her voice tone rising and falling as if she were speaking from a swing. She's lovely to listen to. She surprises me as she lists the many activities in which she participates.

"If I were to list all the things that I do, you would be mortified," she says, expecting people to be surprised by her busy schedule. "I am on the board of directors for a major nonprofit organization. I've been on a governing board for midwifery for a long time and am just now getting off. I was on the grievance committee, on the rule-writing committee, and sat on the committee to write the standards of care for Texas midwives. I was the chairperson of the legislative committee for the bill we just wrote and passed down at the legislature last session," she says.

Without a moment's pause, she shifts her attention to her personal life. "I have four kids, ages twenty-four, twenty-one, seventeen, and twelve." Then back to her professional life, "I'm past vice-president of the midwifery board. They've done most of the legislative work. It's a hotbed of activity. There's always something going on with legislation with midwives."

Again without pause, G.B. continues, "I started a mother's support group in Austin nine years ago that now has nine chapters. I'm an active member of the very first one and mentor new groups that are starting. I'm a midwifery instructor for an oriental medicine school in Austin. And finally, I've taught yoga for more than twenty years."

G.B. oversees about forty to fifty births per year. Besides her midwifery activities, she owns her own business, running a quilting shop in Wimberly, where she teaches classes, makes and sells her own work, and networks with other craft people.

Why and how she manages all this will become clear as her story unfolds. What I can say right now is that life hasn't overtaken her. She's knows what she's doing and continually makes choices to keep a reasonable balance for herself. It may seem frenetic to others, but it serves as a channel for her innately high activity level. She knows when to pull back and has the emotional strength to do just that—like recently leaving the midwifery board so that she could be more effective behind the scenes with legislation.

G.B.'s Background

Raised in Chicago, G.B. sees herself as part of a typical Midwest Irish Catholic-English family. "I drew heavily even as a small child on what I perceived as the courage of the Irish people," she says. "I used to think, 'I am Irish, I am tough, and it is a gift. I'm going to make it.'"

That's the upside of her Irish heritage. The downside, she says, involves what she calls "an intense familial history with alcoholism two or three generations back."

With a younger brother and an older sister, G.B. was introduced to drugs at age twelve when she was offered half of a "purple pill," an amphetamine, if she would iron all of her daddy's shirts.

"She'd give me this big pile of laundry, and I'd iron for hours," G.B. recalls. "This was 1965 and nobody really understood the potential for addiction and damage. They were called 'pep pills' then. I believe my mother's intent was not to hurt me. It was fairly innocent, but she did have severe addiction problems.

"My ADD comes through her line. We were at war from the time I was little." Head nodding as she sensitively reviews the plight of her mother, G.B. comments, "I think she was an extremely sensitive person trying to numb herself to life. She was a teenage mom in the fifties, graduated from high school, and never had the means or power to go beyond that. She was a dreamer. Her bedroom contained a pullout couch that made into a bed and bookshelves with lots and lots of books. She had an encyclopedia, history books, and pain. I know she wanted to be educated. She wanted to live in a big, beautiful house and, instead, she married a Dagwood, a 'putz.'"

Much less clear about her father, she mostly recalls the violence he brought into the home. He had alienated himself from his family by the time G.B. would have gained insight into him. However, she explains how both parents contributed to the family violence with her mother often provoking the fights.

"My father physically beat my mother a number of times and beat us under the direction of my mother frequently. My childhood was not a happy one," she recalls.

G.B. was hesitant to speak about her childhood initially. And no wonder, with a history of violence, drugs, alcohol, and being called "stupid." Who would want to remember that? But in trying to understand her, I gently persist.

"So what kind of little kid were you?" I ask. G.B. answers by looking back at both the negative parts of her childhood—the childhood she remembers clearly—and the positive parts, which she has uncovered only through hypnosis as an adult. Her experience with hypnosis has had a profound effect on many aspects of G.B.'s life.

"Through a combination of my environment, with my parents and at school, I felt totally dumb, bona fide stupid, by the time I was ten. But through hypnosis, I discovered that I was the happiest, most exuberant, irrepressible, totally irrepressible, child up until eight, when my life really started to sour.

"My mother called me a 'dirt magnet.' My parents would liken me to Pigpen in the cartoon," G.B. recalls. "Also, the drinking and violence at home had increased. My father shot a gun in the house once and made my mother believe he had shot himself. She took us all outside where we sat on the porch until the police came and took us away. Mother tried to leave with us one time, but my father came out with a sledge hammer and broke all of the windows in the car.

"My family's form of affection was to tease and chide you in public, especially when we were with the extended family, which was often. I remember humiliation being a regular feeling. For instance, when I began menstruating, it was announced at a family dinner with lots of snickers and remarks: 'Oh, that explains why she acts that way!' It was quite difficult to understand at twelve years old. I felt like an alien in my family."

As early as age eight or nine, she began to have poor reports coming home from school. "They weren't very growth producing," G.B. says, using her typical form of understatement. "I heard teachers tell my parents, 'She was smart, but she always has these behavior problems,' which meant she wasn't smart any more, and she also still has behavior problems."

"What kind of a problems?" I ask.

G.B. tells it this way. "I was probably in the fourth grade when a teacher put on some African music. I got out of my chair and started dancing. I didn't hear her tell me to sit down. By the time I finally heard her, she was raging and, of course, I got sent down to the principal. That kind of trouble."

Until the middle of fourth grade, G.B. was mostly an A student. She feels it was the home factors that "made my brain blow a fuse. When you're little and you can't integrate 'Why is this person yelling at me? Why is this violent thing happening?'— you turn off part of your brain."

Certainly the abuse caused a great deal of stress and no doubt contributed to her school learning problems, which took the form, according to G.B., of "functional dyslexia." G.B. probably is physiologically dyslexic, but in addition, the severe emotional stress in her life exacerbated both her ADD and other learning differences.

But fourth grade is also the time that many very bright children begin to lose ground because of their ADD wiring and learning differences such as dyslexia. They can no longer manage to cover their weaknesses as the complexity of their assignments increases. When these children are constantly being flooded with educational expectations that don't fit the way they are wired, that conflict begins to leave its marks of self-doubt on previously happy children—children who can learn, but not in the way they are being taught. As a result, G.B. began to fail—like so many others.

She dropped out of high school at fifteen, never getting her GED. "We'd lost our house, everything, and went to live with our grandmother. It was traumatic. We moved from the country into the city where the education was very different, and I was way behind. I never caught up. I started acting out with drugs and alcohol. I moved out of my house at fifteen, then went back and left again at seventeen. I probably left three times before I left for good."

It's not surprising that G.B. was pregnant out of wedlock by nineteen. In explanation, with a clear voice, she says, "That pregnancy gave me the chance to realize I needed to drastically change who I was. I was addicted to drugs. I was drinking alcohol on a daily basis, big time, and was pretty much a mess living on the streets of Chicago. I would go from one person's house to another or sleep in the park.

"But then I got pregnant. I had to decide if I was going to stay pregnant or not. I took quantities of drugs the night I was trying to decide. And I got a very clear message: I needed to go on and figure what life is about.

"A friend of mine said, 'Go to this ashram in Tucson, Arizona. People wear white there and talk about peace, and they'll take good care of you.'" She drove south with a friend and stayed in Tucson for a month before eventually moving into the ashram. "I started doing yoga and meditation daily, and I met my husband. I shed who I was," she says.

Over the years, G.B. has worked both on her learning problems and on the emotional residue left by her early life experiences. Sweetly, she confides, "My husband tells me every day, 'If you died today, you did it, you made it, you hit the summit, you made the top of the mountain because you broke the cycle of your childhood.'

"It was hard. There was no affectionate touching when I was growing up. I had to learn to physically touch my children, learn to breast feed and acknowledge their feelings and it was really, really hard work."

Watching the small woman sitting opposite me, I could feel both her strength—the strength of having overcome so much—and the delicacy that makes it such a miracle she survived at all. Yet some of her life-saving endurance was rooted in the creative interests she had in early childhood. The creative, ADD style of brainwiring that made her so sensitive also opened the doors for her survival.

She says, "I made little things. I drew and painted and sewed. I was always in my room reading about making pottery and woodcarving. My grandfather had a lathe in the basement. I used to go down there and turn wood on the lathe. I'd just stand there for hours and feel the wood. I completely redid the furniture in my bedroom. I'd be up there for days just making things. Making things gave me a feeling of completion. It made me feel 'I can make things happen.'"

I found myself wondering how in the world she was able to become a midwife without having a high school diploma? And how has she been able to be involved in all the legislative writing and board work without higher education?

I hesitated even to ask her these questions, because I felt certain that she would feel a sting of inadequacy when I did. But they were questions that were important because she represents the professional who can learn a set of skills without necessarily having gone through formal education.

Those doors, increasingly closed to people with ADD, serve no constructive purpose. They cheat the world of the availability of potential professional talent. Required testing unnecessarily restricts people, blocking them from fulfilling their potential— even though they are able to do the job for which they're being tested.

G.B.'s reaction to not having a GED exemplifies the pain suffered by many people. Summing it up in one sentence, she says, "It's on my mind all the time. Getting a GED will be the last hurrah. When I do that I will feel like I have reached the summit. I can put my past to rest."

Solemnly, she continues, "But I feel terror thinking about taking the GED test. The preparation books are around the house. We use them in my seventeen-year-old son's home schooling. I study them when I can. But my heart races and my palms sweat when I pick up a book to study.

"Part of me feels like a fraud even though no one knows I don't have a high school education. People wouldn't guess. And part of me says, 'Who cares?' I've known some stupid Ph.D.s with no sense and many physicians who do a much poorer job than a midwife with a normal birth. But I still need to do the GED thing for me."

I bet she will, perhaps not long from now.

Nine years ago, at age thirty-five, G.B. decided she needed a "badge of honor" to validate her capabilities. So she registered for training as an Emergency Medical Technician (EMT).

"That was a pivotal time in my life," she says. "You see, it was only four years earlier that I realized I had a learning disability. I was on a search to find out why I felt so stupid. And I wanted to do something about it because I had no self-esteem." After a slight pause she adds for emphasis, "Zero."

Reading was hard, but she creatively developed ways to get through her EMT course work. She developed flash cards to quiz herself—and soon her classmates wanted to buy them. G.B. says, "These were vital because they replaced intricate concepts with single words.

"I was too embarrassed to ask adults for help or advice, so I always got my kids to help me. I would give them the answers to my tests and make them sit with me for hours to review," she says. "When I was learning to speak Spanish, I would always seek out children to talk to because I knew they wouldn't laugh at me."

I also wondered how she has managed to do all the legislative work she has done over the years. "It's intuitive," she says, "and I have grit. I think people depend on me for that grit. I can sit with three House of Representatives members and their aides and two representatives from the Department of Health and at least act like I'm not afraid."

However, there's one more secret that G.B. has to pass on. She puts it this way. "I also rely heavily on my passion for what I believe. I have helped so many families have safe, fulfilling birth experiences that I've drawn strength from them when I have to face the lions.'" That's part of G.B.'s secret.

With a smile on her lips, G.B. says, "The irony of my life is that I have been led so deeply into the world of paper and words. I never could have done that until I was hypnotized and calmed down. When I first started being on those ad hoc committees after EMT school, I had to consciously use the suggestions that the hypnotist gave me. I realized at that time how much of my life was an act of courage. I now have an understanding after EMT school and the legislative work. I can make it through anything.

"It's pretty amazing. Yep, I think what I have now is an understanding of myself that I can figure out anything if I'm just patient with myself. I'm not stupid. I just have had to figure out a different way to approach the world."

Then she adds what all of us who compensate for our weak areas know: "I always depend on other people to do the detail work. I rely on others to read really carefully. Then I listen very carefully to what they say."

G.B.'s husband of twenty-four years, who is now battling multiple sclerosis, is one person she turns to for "the detail work." She says, "He's very analytical. I depend on him to ground me. He is a constant presence, a practical person who definitely gets everyone up on time and ready for school. He makes sure everybody does their homework and sees that the money gets in the bank.

"My husband is my hero. He stood under me, in front of me, and behind me. My healing would never have happened without him. He's the one. I wouldn't have made it without him."

Their relationship has not always been smooth, however. "The first ten years were rough as he constantly pointed out my mistakes," she says. "But I was very reckless and not very mindful. We had a lot of kids, and I had a lot to get over emotionally.

"Now, though, he is extremely apologetic for the way he was. He'd had a very traditional upbringing," she says. "He'd been raised carefully. He knew how to be careful. He'd gone to college, had been a good student in school, one of those upper-middle-class people, and he knew right where my weaknesses were.

"We're beyond that now. It's not part of our relationship any more. As a matter of fact, he's just crazy for me now. He's just in awe of what I've accomplished."

For both G.B. and her husband, religion plays an important role in life. She explains, "We're both Sikhs, but he's more traditional than I am. He wears a turban and is a very devotional man, getting up at four o'clock in the morning to do prayers, read, and meditate in a very sweet way, not in a fanatical way. He's unconditionally devoted to his family, extremely emotional, and very romantic, very right-brained in terms of love and God and numerology—very emotional stuff. Since his multiple sclerosis has developed we've kind of switched places. Now that I've done some healing, it's his turn."

Many of G.B.'s clients now see her as saintly, peaceful, and angelic. She does have that air about her. Though no longer talking about her childhood on a regular basis, she says she quickly sets her clients straight, by saying, "Let me tell you some things about myself."

G.B. explains, "In the course of prenatal care, a trust is built between the midwife and the client. Hour-long visits allow for discussions of not only physical discomforts but also emotional or familial turmoil typical to pregnancy. Often women don't realize how much chaos is inherent to pregnancy and marriage. They are embarrassed to divulge the 'darker' sides of their lives. This is when it is helpful to explain my past, that we all have flaws and challenges.

"Then I'll talk about going to Cook County jail because of drug and alcohol use. I don't do it for shock value, but to tell people, 'You can find a way. My way may not be your way. We each have problems, even people you think don't have them. You can find a way.'"

When I First Met G.B.

When I was looking for raw wool to make into wallhangings, an acquaintance gave me the name and phone number of G.B. Khalsa. It took me a few weeks to make my way to Wimberly, a small town southwest of Austin, but when I did, I was in for a pleasant surprise.

Not only did I find the raw wool I wanted, but the shop owner and I instantly began to talk—talk about all kinds of things: yarn, natural dyes, basket weaving, and creative quilting. We became caught up in completing each other's sentences, exploring in rapid fire the similarities and differences between us.

When I mentioned that I was writing a book about successful people who are constructed in the ADD way, she told me she's ADD and dyslexic, too. While we were talking, I found myself thinking about this wonderful woman I'd just met. I admired her. I felt drawn to her compassion and creativity. And finally I realized what a successful life she has managed to carve out for herself despite ADD, dyslexia, and tough beginnings.

What more could I ask for in a definition of "success?" Recognizing what I'd found, I asked her right there at our first meeting whether she would be willing to let me interview her. She agreed instantly, saying that she would do anything to help others.

How G.B. Envisions the Future

G.B. has lived most of her life being strongly affected by her past. Now she is living in the present a great deal of the time—having put much of her past to rest. The future is still beyond her, she says, at least in terms of planning for it.

"As a child, and even into adulthood, I had this perception of myself as not being able to complete things. I now recognize that I have always had an incredible love of life, a natural curiosity that led me to want to explore everything—to touch, see, feel everything."

Reflecting back to when she was hypnotized, she continues, "Through hypnosis, I saw in great visual detail that I, as a child, was moving, skipping, flitting from one area to another with absolute radiance. Now I realize that I have always just wanted to embrace so much of life—to taste it all. But the stumbling block has been that I didn't know how to do it—taste life, embrace it—like everyone else."

But again, her experience with hypnotism provided a way. "I was helped to remember that essential love of life that can carry me through life. I don't have to do it like everyone else. I realized that my love drove me to learn things that by regular standards I should not have been able to learn. The hardest part, though, has been admitting my shortcomings to instructors who I perceive as having the natural gift, 'brains.' I have often been ashamed of how hard I have had to work to understand. I felt others had done something awfully good at some point because they had been 'given' this marvelous gift of intelligence."

What I hope for in G.B.'s future is that she will fully and totally see and know herself as I see her. That will be her gift to herself and to others.

G.B. also wants to pass on what's she's learned about parenting. She says, "If your child is not consistently doing well, seek out other forms of education. There are more educational options than ever before, certainly more than in the 1950s. Don't let finances, time, or distance be obstacles. Many alternative schools have scholarships and work programs for parents to supplement tuition. If distance is a problem, carpool."

She continues, "If you cannot find a school you like, consider home schooling or co-oping with other home schoolers. I feel very strongly about this because I feel that if you can come through your childhood with self-esteem, it will be the tool to assist you in any endeavor you choose.

"It took me thirty-five years to regain the self-esteem that was stolen from me at age seven by mainstream society's opinions. Do not let teachers label your child. Often they do not have the education to do this, to recognize a child who truly needs professional help. Do not listen to neighbors or friends who label your child."

Finally, G.B. asks that we all listen to what we say to children and how we say it. "Yelling and screaming hurts children and all sensitive people. And are not all people sensitive until scarred?

"When we attend to our own feelings and frustrations, doors will no longer be slammed to vent anger and raised voices will no longer shatter self-esteem. Let us all listen.

"The answer is not to get the child back to normal, make the child a 'regular kid.' You probably have an above-average kid already, and you're blessed. You may have to change your perspective of that child to appreciate and love her."

The light that shines from G.B. is truly the light of a healed healer who has overcome a tough beginning, successfully breaking the cycle previously passed from generation to generation. Her inspirational comments are for all to take advantage of. She knows!

Works For and Against G.B.

G.B.'s tremendous tenacity and resilience have helped her survive and also helped her keep alive her tremendous love of learning. She's learned to reframe her image of herself, and she's figured out how to function in a world that doesn't much fit her. Stick-to-it-iveness, an often overlooked ADD trait, results from being a kinesthetic learner, a person who learns by doing. Life is the schoolhouse of the ADD person who learns by living. Life keeps signing us up for semester after semester of classes so we can keep learning. That adds up to toughness and, in the long run, success.

G.B. can do many, many things, and she can almost do them

all at the same time. That ability is a gift that comes with her ADD. She switches gears easily from one activity to the next.

"I have no trouble going from one thing to another," she says. "As a midwife I have to be able to get a phone call and immediately do a mental inventory of twenty-five things at one time.

"I ask myself, 'Do I need to be there right now? Do I need to give the birthing mother any instructions?' Then I say to myself, 'I need to get my equipment,' which leads to more questions. 'Do I have everything in my bag? Are my children where they need to be? Do I pick up my children from school today? Did I put my money in the bank last night, because I won't be able to leave the birth?' I have to have the instant ability to shift gears."

Yet, ironically, just sitting with G.B. for a few minutes has a calming effect. Naturally, the years of meditation and yoga contribute to her quiet demeanor, but in addition, she has been able to take her ADD sensitivity and turn it around so that others benefit from it. How nice!

In contrast to these positive attributes of ADD, when I asked G.B. about difficulties associated with ADD, "putting things off," popped right out of her mouth.

"I have more confidence now than ever before that I can figure things out. I just don't have the habit of thinking of things ahead of time," she says. "For instance, if I am to go to one of these legislative writing sessions, I do all my paperwork the night before. That's not enough time to digest it, not for me, because I don't read well. I make mistakes when I'm reading. When I pay my bills I make many mistakes. When I make out my bank deposit I make mistakes. I get thinking about something else like, how proud I am of myself for having gotten to the bank on time."

But self-talk helps her make headway in overcoming her self-doubt. "I say to myself, 'Yeah! Oh, that's fine. I'm at the bank.' I'm thinking how wonderful I am that I'm finally catching on to how to be responsible, to be like everyone else."

G.B. joyfully raises and lowers her voice, expressing an auditory dance of delight as she finishes saying, "Ten years ago I wouldn't have done any of this. I would have been bouncing checks all over the place."

G.B. has one major task yet to accomplish: She needs to admit to herself that she is as capable as she is. But with a serious look on her face, she responds, "I can't get to that. My mind can't think that is possible. That's going to take a lot of work. That wouldn't come naturally to me to automatically assume I was going to do it right. I'll have to work on that."

Mother Teresa had recently died when I was interviewing G.B., and I commented on her ability to see the best in everyone. I knew that G.B.'s own belief system supports this, and I knew that the serious look on her face was her own struggle to live what she believes.

"You know, I can see the best in my children and in other people, but haven't been able to see the effect in myself."

G.B.'s struggle stems partly from the abuse she suffered as a child and partly from being wired in a way that differs from the accepted model for excellence in this culture. With her tenacity, though, I know she will continue to work on seeing herself with as much charity as there is in how she sees others.

Fortunately, G.B.'s own self-worth is in good hands. The outcome is guaranteed. I can hardly wait until G.B. discovers the truth about herself.

WHAT G.B. WANTS YOU TO KNOW

Inside of you there is a miracle.

What you love to do is who you are; do what you love to do.

Have the courage to be yourself; your uniqueness is your gift.

Bill Hayes

You have to make peace with your past. BH

And he's certainly a living representative of having done so. LW

Laid back. Of all the people I know, this description fits Bill Hayes the best. It's not that his affect is flat or that he seems straight-laced, but rather that he is mellow. When I talk with him, I always feel listened to and responded to. I know I have his attention. He comes across as a warm, empathic, and at times playful person. I know this from the lift of his eyebrow, a softening of his glance, or the nod of his head rather than through lots of words or big gestures.

On the one hand, I experience Bill as a very responsible one-has-to-pay-the-consequences-of-one's-behavior kind of person. On the other hand, I see a broad-minded, gently adventurous man who quietly negotiates a pathway between these two ways of being.

When I ask him for a representative reflection of his ADD, he says, "I probably make decisions quickly because I don't like to make choices. I've had to learn to live with that. There are consequences when you make bad choices not based on any thought process or evaluation."

There it is. Bridging the distance between the tendency to be impulsive and spontaneous. His challenge is to build a pathway that allows him to use his good thinking mind to process and evaluate information so that he can make choices that please him. Those pathways must connect with the world in which he's chosen to live. Bill is well on his way to doing that.

He quickly confides an ADD experience from ten years ago, when he and his family moved to Valparaiso, Indiana, where they currently live. Bill was working then, as he is now, at a steel mill. The company had transferred him several times, so this was not his family's first move.

Like many couples facing a move, Bill and his wife sat down and talked about how much money they had to spend, where the best schools for their children were located, and how far they were willing to drive to work. They had already decided they wanted a home in the city. His wife, the investigator, then went to work and gathered information so that they could make a good decision.

But Bill didn't like any of the houses that fit their parameters. "I just didn't feel comfortable," he explains. So what did he do? He continued to look until he found a house he liked. It was outside the city in a different school district—one they hadn't even considered—and he said, "This is it!"

In retrospect, Bill says, "I work from emotion. My wife is the one who has her feet on the ground. I'm getting better, but I still occasionally struggle with reacting emotionally."

Bill's Background

"I was the first grandchild on my father's side of the family. My two aunts doted on me. They fought over me. They always said I was a chatterbox, always asking questions—so much so that they came to the conclusion that I was probably going to be a doctor, because I was so interested in things." Today he adds with a bit of a chuckle, "That was probably my little hyperactive motor going there."

Some of the ease leaves his voice as he relates how the peace and tranquility of his early surroundings quickly gave way to disruption. His parents fought, even physically, and separated for a time when Bill was in the first grade. At that time, the family lived in a small town outside Pittsburgh. When Bill was a teenager, his family moved into the city.

"I now realize that my father was probably ADD and was quite impulsive. Usually he had two or three jobs," Bill says. "Never having graduated from grade school, he'd gone to work in the steel mill where he did clerical work. He stayed with the mill throughout his work life. But he was also an entrepreneur—someone who gravitated to high-risk jobs—in addition to ones that took him away from home much of the time."

Hesitating for a moment when I ask what kind of high-risk jobs his father held, Bill says his father did police work and worked in a service station. Then he adds, "He got into gambling and bookmaking on the side. Oh, and during the war [World War II] he had an affair. Yes, my dad was probably ADD. He did a lot of crazy stuff.

"I had a lot of resentment toward my dad and have worked hard to get beyond it. It's very important to get beyond the past," Bill says softly.

In contrast to his father, Bill's mother had been raised in a environment where risks were not taken. Though she said she forgave her husband for his affair, "she never let anyone else forget it," Bill says. His parents separated twice, and Bill's two younger brothers are five years apart—the result of their making up. Finally, though, his parents came back together and stayed together until his father died a few years ago.

The trauma from his parents' stress was compounded by Bill's own trouble in school when he repeated the second grade. Even today, you can hear the sadness in his voice for that little boy who felt so miserable.

"It was a real downer having to repeat second grade," Bill says, as if he were looking at himself from a distance. "There was a real unhappiness in a kid who flunked a grade and watched his family being destroyed." After a short hesitation, he adds, "Mother wanted to put me in a foster home, and I didn't want that. I made a terrible scene about the whole thing. I didn't want any part of that."

Apparently Bill's wishes prevailed, so that he was kept at home. Still, he says, "I never worked up to potential. I told myself, 'I can do better than that,' but I didn't do very well. Later, I did go to college, but I was programmed to fail because of my mother's background. She told me, 'You're not going to make it. No one in our family ever went to college.'

"It was like—she predicted the future. I spent three semesters, and she was right. Now I realize that I also ran up against a lot of ADD stuff, like not being able to concentrate or focus my attention on what I was studying."

After dropping out of college as a young man, Bill went to work in the steel mill, like his father, initially doing clerical work for quality control in the technical services department. After four years at the mill, he entered the U.S. Air Force, where he stayed for four years.

In the air force, Bill developed Crohn's disease, a digestive tract disorder that is exacerbated by stress. As a result, he was discharged from the air force slightly earlier than he had planned. After his discharge, Bill returned to work at the steel mill and he's been there ever since. He has risen through the ranks—through servicing accounts and working as a statistician and claims investigator—into management and sales. Five years ago, Bill and his wife decided they didn't want to be moving around any more. It was then that Bill transferred into sales, and he has been managing the steel mill's largest account since then.

Bill married Jeanne when he was thirty-one. Twins were born within two years and eventually he and Jeanne had a third child. Those were stressful years for Bill and Jean. The company moved them several times. He changed jobs within the company, and they found themselves under lots of pressure trying to coordinate careers, child rearing, and keeping a personal life going.

Though he worked hard and tried hard, Bill was nearly fifty years old before the pieces of his life truly began to come together. He was diagnosed with ADD the same way so many other adults are diagnosed—after recognizing their children's ADD symptoms in themselves. When Bill's sons were identified as being ADD, Bill's life, too, took a turn for the better.

He tells it this way: "Jeanne is very intuitive. I did one right thing in this life. I married the person I should have. I married someone to compensate for my weakness. So when our sons came up ADD, Jeanne turned to me and said, 'Maybe that's you, too.'"

"I did what a lot of parents do. I tried my son's Ritalin and Jeanne said, 'My, what happened to you?'"

"I asked her what she meant, and she told me the changes she saw. Jeanne said, 'I think you better go to the doctor.'"

Bill followed that advice and was diagnosed with ADD in 1992. He rejoices in the changes that this diagnosis has brought to his life. He feels that it not only saved his marriage but helped him become the person he has become—a person he feels good about, rather than one who is not living up to his potential.

Bill might not have made it through college directly after high school, but he never gave up. With a remarkable and admirable tenacity, Bill went back to college as an adult and graduated in 1993, almost thirty-five years after he first entered. Like so many other accomplishments in Bill's life, this one came late by some standards. But for Bill—who, like many people with ADD, is a late bloomer—it came at exactly the right time.

"You know, it was just something I needed to finish, and I did," he says with a pleased, gently powerful tone in his voice. "Yes, I finished with the help of medication and understanding of ADD. I self-identified with ADD in 1992 and then was professionally diagnosed later the same year."

The early 1990s were a turning point in Bill's life, with both his ADD diagnosis and his college graduation coming during those years. Yes, he was in his fifties when he was diagnosed with ADD, and, yes, he probably could have avoided a lot of difficulty and unhappiness had he been diagnosed earlier. But it's never too late to begin to truly understand ourselves. And that's certainly one of the most important things I've learned from knowing Bill. His life serves as a remarkable example for all late bloomers.

As a result of his ADD diagnosis—and, according to Bill, as a result of his using medication to treat his ADD—he went from having to go to his office at the steel mill on weekends so that he could study in complete silence to being able to write a philosophy paper one professor described as "writing at a master's level." Before his ADD diagnosis, he'd had to take off some semesters of college, when the stress got too high. During other semesters, he simply stretched himself to cover his daytime job while studying during off hours.

"It was difficult for the family, but I was determined that I had to do it," he says. And in the end, he completed his work for a psychology degree—and feels mighty proud. Talk about perseverance!

Interestingly, Bill's health has improved dramatically since 1992. When he went for his regular Crohn's checkup a year after he had begun to be treated for his ADD, his doctor said, "You don't have any evidence of Crohn's disease. None. Not a trace. None." That was about five years ago and there's still no trace.

More and more often, those of us working in the ADD

community are seeing stress-related conditions like Crohn's disease subsiding when ADD is recognized and managed, and people feel better about themselves. What a wonderful side effect to the identification of this special way of being brainwired.

Part of what is happening here is that a diagnosis of ADD often relieves a tremendous amount of guilt. The ADD individual often believes that if he would just work hard enough, he would be successful. So if he isn't experiencing success, he assumes he just isn't working hard enough—and feels terribly guilty. Also, when people are officially identified as having ADD, they often feel free to get some help—whether that's organizational help, counseling, tutoring—help that gives them a much better chance of living up to their special potential.

Bill, like so many other people, felt a big load come off his shoulders when he was formally identified as being ADD. Finally, he understood what had been causing him trouble. And armed with that information, he could go about getting the help he needed. It didn't really matter that he was in his fiftiess at that time—better late than never.

When I First Met Bill

I first met Bill in 1993 when he was president of the National Attention Deficit Disorder Association and I was on the board of directors. My earliest memories were of a sweet, mild man who smiled somewhat shyly but could also hold tightly to a principle in the face of conflict. I also saw someone who enjoyed the creative process of organizing large events, such as an ADD conference. And, in fact, in addition to his job at the steel mill, Bill has started a small business of his own organizing conferences. Those organizational skills are clearly ones that bring Bill a sense of accomplishment and joy.

As in all groups, there exists diversity within ADD organizations.

Many members of the board that year were ADD, although a few were not. And given the many forms of ADD, and the diversity of personality styles, differences naturally arose periodically. But I never had any doubt that fairness would prevail under Bill's presidential gavel.

After I was no longer a board member, I watched Bill work with other groups. I observed him develop his conference-planning business, and I have come to know him as a friend to whom I can speak candidly. Though we've not spent a lot of time together, we've slowly observed each other's vulnerable sides and rejoiced in one another's strengths. My sense of Bill is that he makes a good and loyal friend—one who will be around for a long time.

Bill sees his life as being divided into two parts: "BM" and "AM": before medication and after medication. And he is adamant about his use of medication to treat his ADD.

Though I'm not against the use of medication and, in fact, see it as absolutely necessary for many people to survive in the educational and work systems as they now stand, I have chosen to work outside the field of medication. My focus is on trying to change the environments that require ADD people to function like non-ADD people. In fact, I do not have much interest in trying to fit into settings that do not honor a person's strengths and natural abilities.

Consequently, it might seem that Bill and I would have a conflict, or at least differences, that would make it difficult to have a mutually respectful relationship. But that is not the case. I respect and admire him and believe I understand a lot about the choices he makes. And I believe he offers me that same respect.

I have to admit that when I first heard Bill say, "BM" and "AM," I cringed. The medicalizing and pathologizing of ADD causes me great pain. Too often, I see people grab the magic bullet of medication and do nothing else to learn to manage the attributes that cause them trouble.

But Bill, in his inimitable fashion, neither judges my position nor touts his own as better; he does not wear his medication usage as a badge. He simply rejoices in the fact that he can more easily and effectively perform some tasks that are extremely valuable to him—tasks that are a necessary part of what he loves to do, such as managing conferences. Bill—who was unable to have any kind of control over his life as a child when he lost the security of his doting aunts, his tight family unit, and the ability to be taught effectively in school—is able to use the framework provided by medication to gain control now.

Listening to him, I also experience the pleasure he gets from working within a system. He doesn't use systems rigidly to wield power over people nor does he demand absolute obedience. He makes use of them to provide supportive structure so that the people within them can reach their goals. Bill enjoys tidying up loose ends. It pleases him to present a smooth-running package where everything has its place.

When something "goes wrong," at a conference for example, he doesn't panic but methodically goes about correcting what's wrong. Soon whatever was amiss has been taken care of and all is again well with the world.

How Bill Envisions the Future

At nearly sixty, Bill looks forty-five. "It's in the genes," he says. But he also notes how many of us who are ADD mature physically more slowly than our non-ADD counterparts. Married at thirty-one, which he describes as "late," he feels he's aged more slowly than many others he knows. "I don't feel or think 'fifty-nine.' It's hard to think about retirement. It'll be quite a transition."

Bill is currently in what I call the "Coming of Age" stage of his life. This is a stage people commonly go through after their ADD is first identified. For many people, this is a time when they are first able to make sense of so many aspects of their lives, and form a new identity in the process. Able to reach his potential perhaps for the first time, Bill is redefining his values, honoring his talents, and loving who and what he is.

Because he's just now "finding" himself, Bill does not have a lot of clearly defined goals for the future.

But when I look at him, I see a man whose future holds, at least in part, the role of teacher. And he is already stepping into that role. Informally, Bill shares his beliefs about ADD in his low-key manner. Without necessarily even meaning to, he reflects the truth that it is never too late to put your life together. His students are often people whose paths he crosses as a part of his conference work. He reaches out to others, sharing his perspective of human nature. Then he adds a topping of his perspectives on the ADD nature of things.

"What I see in the ADD world is a lot of people searching for self-actualization and happiness and all those things that everybody strives for," he says.

He feels, however, that society teaches people the wrong thing. "Rather than looking for perfection within, I have learned to not get too upset or stressed by my imperfections," he says. "Sure, I've learned to a greater degree to develop my talents, interests and passions. But I've also learned to forget my weaknesses. Or, at least, to only work on them to some extent while not getting too excited about them."

Bill is concerned that a lot of ADD people are too focused on themselves and their own pain, so that they don't have room to carry someone else's burden. "I think I'm a giver instead of a taker. I ask very little for myself," Bill says. "There's not a lot that I need. I've been able to understand that I am healed and my burden lightened when I turn my attention and energy toward helping someone else."

His stance is indicative of how far Bill has come, how much

healing he has been able to achieve. He's moved to a place where he's dealt with a lot of his anger about his past. Rather than blaming others for what happened, he's been able to make peace with what happened to him in his own childhood.

"It was hard to let go of stuff, but I think I've done it," he says. Now he passes on his desire that others take responsibility for themselves. And they will in time—as their hurts are healed and they see how they, too, can reach their own potential and be self-responsible.

Looking and feeling young and confident as he does, is it any wonder that Bill is considering going into business for himself full-time and quitting his job at the mill? His eyes glow as he talks about putting on conferences. But they also cloud over a bit when he thinks about leaving the structure of his current job.

"It's a dilemma," says Bill. "I'm doing very well at work handling the company's biggest account and being recognized for it. That's hard to walk away from. But eventually I have to. On the other hand, I need the security of a steady income. But yet, I still have that entrepreneurial spirit that says, 'Be your own boss. Do your thing.' It's a passion to do what I'm doing."

A lot of Bill's rewards come not from monetary sources but from the prestige and admiration he receives. It's easy to hear the pleasure in his voice as he says, "I rejoice in helping others get well."

With sweetness, Bill concludes, "I look forward to spending more time with my wife and having fun—traveling, seeing people we like, and doing the kind of work I want to do."

What Works For and Against Bill

A self-made, emotionally healthy person, Bill is functional and responsible, thanks to the work he's done on himself. Through counseling, reading, self-observation, and the responsible use of medication, he's learned to work with his ADD way of being constructed.

He often gives his wife Jeanne the credit. Bill's zest for life and sweet nature coupled with his wife's firm limits and expectations make a successful outcome for both of them.

Though life-long depression haunted Bill until he began to use medication for ADD, he now has accumulated lots of experience at feeling good. Since his use of medication, he's not had trouble with depression. Realizing that, he says, "I've become religious about taking my meds."

Is it any wonder? Who would want to return to the oppressive feelings of depression? And with his newfound freedom, he is able to use his ADD attributes to his advantage.

A behavior that used to be a liability also helps him now with his depression. Little Bill's "motor mouth" has turned into a very useful ADD-related skill: self-talk.

"I use it a lot to plan my day," he shares. "I question my reasons and motives. I think things through." Talking about feelings and making plans definitely gives Bill a mighty tool to use with depression.

Innocence and trustworthiness, shared by a lot of his ADD peers, are keys to Bill's personality. He communicates trustworthiness and doesn't seem to have a conniving bone in his body. As a result, others respond openly. Even shy people tend to be able to connect to Bill.

His sensitivity, another ADD trait, allows him to "read" what's going on with another person. When he picks up the cue, he waits, he listens, and then he waits some more. Such an enticement draws the speaker out—and the next thing you know, you're talking to him.

Sometimes his innocence and sensitivity work against him, though. The attributes that make him a good and loyal friend also get him into trouble—a common issue for people with ADD attributes. He says, "I'm unrealistic about people. Not holding back at first with someone or not accepting what I do see causes me to fail to look deeper. Then I find out I'm disappointed in the person later. I may find they are not the person I thought they were. Maybe I've already given too much of myself."

He's trying to change that.

"I'm trying to learn to reserve judgment, wait for things to play out instead of jumping right in," he says.

He'll get it, I'm sure. Now Bill is marrying his sensitivity to his desire to have things stable and structured around him. With this bridge in place, he is more able to control situations rather than be controlled by them.

Bill doesn't want or need to control other people. He does, however, benefit from having himself in tow. The result: markedly less frustration. Where previously he was haunted by events and people in chaos, he now can relax, knowing he is in control. He puts it this way. "I'm not going to make a move or do a job that I don't want to do, even if it means not having the job."

Again, Bill partly attributes his current ability to handle complex situations to his use of medication. "Now on my job in sales, I can walk away from some work I'm doing and reconnect with it when I return. That's new behavior for me," he says with pride. "I have things under control because I can prioritize them now. I do the hard things first and use the easy things as a reward. I've learned to not panic, because I've learned you're more effective when you don't."

How did he learn to not panic?

"Well, I understand myself now. I have to go back to medication. That's me. That's not everybody, but it's worked for me. I like being organized and on top of things."

That's the key. Bill really likes being organized. It seems to be an innate part of his personality. So, to be able to work the way he truly wants, not how he thinks he should, Bill gets the help he desires from medication.

As he gains practice with his new behaviors he may or may not find he continues to need medication. It really doesn't matter whether he does or doesn't use it indefinitely. He'll know what is right for him. What is important is that he's taken the time to learn behaviors that have made him able to express successfully his innate talents and identity.

Bill has learned what makes him happy and what doesn't. He listens to himself as well as he listens to others. It behooves us all to follow in Bill's footsteps.

WHAT BILL WANTS YOU TO KNOW

Make peace with your past and let it go.

Self-evaluate.

Be honest with yourself.

Follow through on what you find.

Go at it with all the fervor you have, wherever that takes you, and go for it.

Callie Briggen

You've got to experience there's another way to be, to live, to feel good about yourself. CB

And she's learned how to do this. LW

Callie was one active kid! For as long as she can remember, she has expressed herself physically. Take the time she and her dad were waiting for her sister and mother to come out from a piano lesson. Five-year-old Callie was in the back seat of the car pushing the cigarette lighter in and out. Alert and inquisitive, she saw that it was a bright red color.

Knowing that it was hot, knowing what it was for, she stuck her thumb right on it nevertheless. She tried real hard to keep still, because she'd already learned to keep a lot of her pain to herself. But it quickly became obvious that something was wrong.

Callie's dad said, "Why did you do that?"

Even today, Callie asks herself the same question she asked that day, "Why did I do that?"

Quickly, as if to verify that she was "out of control," Callie tells me about another incident, also when she was five.

"I was afraid to get into the kiddie section of the neighborhood swimming pool. But there I stood, right by the pool," she says. "The next thing I knew I'd picked up a wavy wooden flutterboard, sailed it at some other kids playing in the pool, and knocked the two front teeth out of one of the 'trespassers.'" She finishes by saying, "There wasn't any thought." In her mind she sees her action as proof that she was "out of control."

Now fifty-five and a well-respected librarian in upper New York state, Callie no longer throws flutterboards or presses her thumb against cigarette lighters—but she definitely still lives life with exuberance and curiosity. She has a wide-eyed look of wonder on her round face, making her appear years younger than her actual age.

Just yesterday I received a set of pictures of her mountain cabin in upstate New York, not far from where she lives. Callie is helping to build this cabin—hammering in nails regardless of the effect on her own nails. In the picture, she's peeking over the top of an extremely steeply pitched roof, many feet above the highest workman, who is securing logs in place. I couldn't for the life of me figure out how she got up there or what was keeping her up there. So I just inhaled deeply, realizing that I would probably have heard if she hadn't made it down.

Callie is a woman with a definite zest for living. But it's a zest that was dormant for far too long. For years, Callie was depressed, drawing as little attention to herself as she could. During those many years, she suffered from far too many emotional stresses to be relaxed and exuberant. Only with the discovery and identification of her ADD at about age fifty has she been able to blossom again. Although she's still quiet at times, more and more often she's enjoying the little "dickens" who for so long got pushed deep inside herself so that she could stay out of trouble. Now a gentle balance is unfolding.

Callie's Background

As the youngest of four children, Callie always felt very small in a large household of people who were all bigger than she. To some extent, she still feels that way—she tips in at only five feet tall. One sister is six years older, and two half brothers are thirteen and eighteen years her senior.

"I felt kind of alone," she says rather soulfully.

Besides her birth order making it tough for her, when Callie was two her sister fell from a horse, suffering a severe head injury that required a lot of parental focus and travel for treatments. Feelings of loneliness surround Callie as she remembers her sister and dad being gone. "The house was very empty," she says. "My best friend was my fifteen-year-old half brother. I was always in trouble; he was a pain in the rear end, being a teenager. I think that kind of bonded us."

Callie had a lot of "things," not people, in her life. She often played by herself with stuffed animals and blocks. She made tea parties and spent considerable time playing with an old iron that would "shock the living daylights" out of her. She says, "I guess I thought it wouldn't. Then I would plug it in, and it would shock me again."

But her next comment clarifies the reason for her fascination with the iron. Callie tells me, "We had a lady who would come to do housework. I would hang with her down in the basement, and she taught me how to iron everybody's handkerchiefs. It became my job to iron them. I looked forward to that." The cleaning lady was one of the few people who ever gave Callie any real attention. Is it any wonder then that little Callie continued to play with that iron?

She continues her story about her childhood. "I would fantasize that I was in one of the books I was reading. I would walk around the neighborhood pretending I was surrounded by the Bobbsie twins and imagine a whole scene in my mind.

"As I got older, I played with two girls and one boy who lived near me. We were always in fights. All of our mothers were industriously involved in community work. They didn't play with us or provide us with supervised activities. So we went out into the neighborhood and created our own entertainment. Another child, James, who lived near us was the brunt of considerable nastiness. Rather than being compassionate about the fact that he was overprotected by a seriously mentally ill mother, we made him the scapegoat for all our childhood frustrations.

"We felt his mother's mental illness was a mark against him. We teased him about the undershirts and sweaters he was made to wear on hot summer afternoons when the rest of us were running under the hose in our bathing suits.

"I was a real tomboy, just an incredible tomboy, and my mother called me 'the Hellion,'" Callie confides. "But I was little and had blond, curly hair that made me look so cute that it was hard for other grown-ups to believe the reputation I had."

To explain her reputation further, Callie continues to tell about her relationship with James. "You see, the other kids talked negatively about James, but I was usually the one that came through with the good old physical whatever-it-was, whether it was pinning James down or taunting him.

"For example, one day we had chased James up to his house. The housekeeper caught us and stopped and looked at the four of us. James was trying to tell her what happened. She said, 'Oh you can't tell me that little girl with the blond curls is being mean to you!' He looked at me with a chill in his eyes and responded, 'She's the worst one.'

"I was only five or six at the time. I felt awful. This was reinforced by my sister, who called me 'the bad seed.'"

Still with a sense of questioning in her voice, Callie says, "It baffled everybody—and me, too. I still wonder, 'Why did I do such things?'"

I wondered when Callie's behavior changed, because she's certainly not a "bad seed" now. Neither is she ruthless. In fact, she's relatively quiet and low key, and it's difficult now to believe she would have been so mean to another child. The answer came as she told me about being kept in a "little" school when all of her classmates went on to another school. It happened in second grade.

"For the first time in my life I was the biggest person anywhere. I had an excellent teacher and a very free environment. I was given things to do that I could do. My teacher liked me. I wasn't 'bad' there," she says.

Callie was raised from the age of three in a suburban neighborhood by upwardly mobile parents. Her father was a dentist who moved to an upscale neighborhood after he became an oral surgeon, and Callie found herself surrounded by status symbols. She says "My father was very ostentatious with what he could afford, but we were probably the poorest of everybody there, and we had the least fancy background."

The mother she knew was quite different from the one her sister experienced. Apparently before Callie was born, her mother had been very social and a musician, had entertained a lot, was the live wire of the parties she gave, and was generally an outgoing, active person. In contrast, Callie knew her as someone who didn't go out much, didn't shop, stopped driving, had become phobic, and rarely spent time with women friends.

Why, I wondered, was Callie's mother so different after her birth? The answer came without my needing to ask. Callie says, "My father did all the shopping and often took me with him. I spent tons of time with him in the car and heard all of his stories about when he was a little boy and about his college.

"But he also told me I had not been a wanted child, that if there had been birth control, I would have never been born. I don't think he meant it in a mean way, but I grew up feeling I was a mistake. I learned my mother was very unhappy, wanted to abort me, and the only reason she didn't was because no room was available in the hospital during wartime."

We can only speculate that Callie's mom, probably ADD, felt overwhelmed and trapped with four children. Desperate, having lost her freedom and hope for her own self-expression, she dove within herself, shutting down her feelings to a life of depression and fear, as so many women of her day experienced.

Callie's maternal grandfather also expressed ADD-style attributes. She describes him clearly. "He had a million different jobs. He was very inventive. He would create something and live off it for a little while. Then he'd run out of money," she says. "My grandfather loved to play cards, drink, and hoot and holler. My mother was precocious herself but was embarrassed at his behavior—as he and his wife would have money one minute and not the next. Because her parents ran out of money, my mother had to leave her college studies of music to go home and support the family. No wonder she became neurotic!"

Callie and her mother both seemed to be accident-prone. The die was cast for them with quick movements, stress, and having been told, "You're an accident waiting to happen."

To describe her situation, Callie explains, "I understand how my mother kept getting hurt. You go to get a glass out of the cupboard, and your mind wonders what's in the refrigerator. Then you take your eyes off the glass you are holding and blindly whack it against the cupboard door."

In fifth grade, Callie had decided to become a librarian because she loved to read. But then she read a book about a girl who befriended a neighbor boy who was blind and, as she tells it, "I became fascinated by the blind bit and eventually majored in special education."

She went directly to college after high school—even though she hated school. She went to college because that was what was expected of her. But it was difficult for her from the very beginning.

"It would take me forever to do schoolwork. I would do homework for hours and hours and hours," she says. "I would sit down in my chair, I'd get up, I'd move around, I'd get the work wrong, I'd double-check it, I'd spend three hours trying to get it. It was awful."

She also endured a lonely college life. Living in the dorm, studying all the time, and constantly feeling scared to death that she'd be found out to be a total dunce made her feel wretched. Ironically, though, she graduated magna cum laude.

After college, Callie taught for one year as an itinerant special education teacher and then married. Again having trouble doing more than one thing at a time, she quit her job so that she could concentrate on being a wife. Callie stayed home to raise her two daughters for eight years, and they benefited from the time she spent with them. But life was stressful for two reasons. First, Callie found it hard to organize the running of her house efficiently.

"To put on a simple dinner party," she says, "might mean I would end up having to go to the grocery store five or more times, forgetting something each time."

Second, she was called back to teaching blind kids. "I remember when the call came," Callie says. "I was asked whether I'd be willing to put in a couple of days a week—as a favor? The district had no itinerant teacher.

"I was excited. It was neat to think about being in a professional mode again. But before long, I kicked into taking forever to prepare lessons and reports, only now I had two kids, a husband, and a part-time job that became a full-time job for me. It took that long for me to get done what others did more quickly. As a result, my husband got mad. It was tough."

Callie worked part-time for five years before she and her

husband bought a house. Then they ran out of money, and she had to get a full-time job immediately, so she tried her hand at factory work. "Lack of concentration made me less than the best factory worker," she explains.

"As if to save me, the special education folks called asking me to work again. I wasn't happy, though. I didn't look forward to the same visual 'stims' [visual stimulation exercises] with these multiply handicapped kids—not getting more reaction. I had to do the same things in the same way day after day after day, or the kids got confused. But I loved them [the kids]—so I gritted my teeth, all the time feeling very bad."

With her marriage falling down around her, she decided she either had to drop the marriage or go back to school and get a master's degree. She did neither. "Instead I wound up being a part-time cashier at a hardware store. Now that was something!" Callie exclaims.

"People would ask me, 'Don't you get bored there?' No way," Callie says. "I had to work so hard getting through a transaction without making a mistake that I couldn't be bored. Every time a customer came up, adrenaline would kick in. It became a question of 'How can I do this?' It was a kind of puzzle I had to solve.

"Eventually through attrition I became head cashier. It was funny," Callie says with a laugh. "I would train these gals who scanned the store looking for guys, could cashier up a storm, and have a conversation all at the same time. In contrast, I had worked there five or six years needing to focus non-stop to be able to do the job correctly."

Again the thought of going back to school seemed like a solution. "I figured going back to school to get a master's degree in library science would be a breeze after cashiering," Callie told me. "Not so! I truly had no idea that going back to school in my forties was going to be just like it had been the first time around. After all, I was motivated. I felt I could do it, I was in a different spot in my life. I had been a teacher. I knew all these things. Wrong!" she exclaims.

"I was just floored to find I didn't feel one whit different at forty-five. I felt worse. We sat for three hours at a time in class. The accuracy, the detail, the methodicalness of a lot of the work I had to do as a librarian was difficult. My classmates did the same work that I did, got the same grades, and had a life."

Divorced by the time she finished her master's degree, she took a job as outreach librarian eight years ago. It's still hard at times, but Callie is doing a great job. She enjoys a warm rapport with her co-workers and those who work for her. Her boss is a blessing, valuing what Callie can bring to her position while minimizing Callie's areas of weakness. She expects quality results but does not require a rigid program or schedule. So Callie has the freedom to develop her own way of doing things.

Callie enjoys the companionship of a few select friends, has a good relationship with her two grown daughters, and is expanding her interests, such as building the small log cabin on the property she obtained three years ago. But, perhaps most important, Callie is now comfortable with herself. I might even say she likes herself—no mean feat!

When I First Met Callie

One day in 1992, the phone rang while I was sitting at my home computer writing a workbook about managing ADD. It was Callie Briggen. She had found me from the resource list at the end of my first book on ADD. She told me she was a librarian and had found the book while working.

In the book, she said, she found herself.

From reading the book, Callie was sure she was ADD, although she had never been formally evaluated. She asked if I could evaluate her over the phone. Although it was something I had not done before, I thought, why not? I could get the information long-distance just as readily as I could in person. I have a trained ear from working in talk radio three hours a day, five days a week, for seven years. I have thirty years of counseling experience behind me. I could do this responsibly. And so I agreed to the long-distance evaluation.

First, I sent Callie a written evaluation form to fill out, to which I added my notes. Frankly, I was impressed that she was able to fill it out, because it meant spending a lot of time doing paperwork—not an activity usually relished by ADD folks. Either her motivation was incredibly high or she spent a lot of time on it; probably both.

There was something in her voice that was beguiling as she asked for my help. Yes, I could tell she was hurting a lot, was agitated and depressed. But I also could tell she had strength. That's what I banked on, being able to connect with her strength. And I wasn't wrong.

Callie and I worked well together long-distance. "I felt the connection immediately," she says. "Confident that we were on the same page, I allowed fifty years' worth of shame-based defenses to fall away. The therapist with whom I was working at that time was very supportive. She and Lynn conferred by phone as well—each adding to a composite evaluation."

At the time, I was criticized by some of my peers for taking on Callie's evaluation long-distance. Nevertheless, I stood my ground at that time and still stand by this process as a perfectly legitimate alternative to face-to-face evaluations. Sadly, some professionals do not understand that these evaluations can be accurate without all kinds of testing and rigorous notation in a traditional setting. What I understand now is that those professionals do not have the necessary auditory and sensory/feeling skills to conduct nontraditional evaluations. But that doesn't mean those evaluations cannot or should not be done by someone who is adequately equipped to do them.

And I do mean that the person doing the evaluation must be adequately equipped. This is not a situation in which a lay person can read one book on ADD and start evaluating or "diagnosing" ADD over the phone. It takes just as long to understand and gain a professional level of control using auditory, sensory/feelings-based cues as it does with a linear, empirical approach. The intuitive person's data bank must also be filled with information and experience and be tested and retested over time. But it's a comparable, parallel approach to working with people.

Interestingly, during the last few years, telephone "coaching" has become accepted as a perfectly legitimate way to help people with ADD. A less expensive and less formal procedure than traditional therapy or counseling, coaching is a nondirective process in which a trained "coach" provides information and encouragement to the person learning to cope with ADD. Although I was criticized for it at the time, I see my telephone work with Callie and others as a precursor to the now widely accepted practice of telephone coaching.

In any case, thank goodness Callie was able to make use of our process to begin her journey to recovery. From the initial identification of her ADD, she gained the courage to contact a physician about medication. Unfortunately, he did not respect my long-distance diagnosis and referred her to a local professional for reevaluation. Numerous appointments and a substantial amount of money later, my initial clinical report was replicated, and medication was prescribed for Callie's ADD.

It took Callie's physicians two years to find the balance of medication that really worked for her. Her medication journey was fraught with the difficulties often faced by people with ADD wiring. Because many physicians are untrained in regard to ADD, they tend to be more comfortable with medicating the depression and anxiety that often accompany ADD than with helping the individual deal with the actual ADD. They often mistakenly identify depression and anxiety as being the under-lying fundamental issues—when in reality they are the result of a person's untrained, uncontrolled ADD. ADD can also create problems in an environment that doesn't fit. If the ADD is first attended to, many symptoms of depression and anxiety either disappear or are greatly reduced.

Finally, though, Callie was provided with a combination of stimulant and other medications that yielded good results for her. And finally she could tell her before-and-after story.

"Before medication, I often felt bombarded by stimuli that came in and filled my head. And my head was already filled with its own stimuli. So when I was trying to work on a task, I felt like I was trying to battle through vegetable soup, trying to get past intervening thoughts, office noise, whatever was happening, whatever emotions were happening—all at the same time," she explains. "There's a distinct change in my performance on and off the medication. The stew, soup, feels different. It dissipates. I can focus on a conversation. I can sit still."

I met Callie in person for the first time at a national adult ADD conference a year after her initial evaluation. We hit it off immediately. A year later, she came to Texas to spend a week integrating the work she'd done over the previous months. We met daily for a couple of hours, focusing on practical skill-building issues and motivational guidance. She participated in hypnotherapy to reframe the beliefs about herself that held her captive to a negative self-image. At the end of the week, she left to start a new chapter of her life, one that might be titled, "Liking Callie."

How Callie Envisions the Future

Callie stands out in my mind as a warrior who has fought a battle with inner self-degradation and dislike. Now she stands on the podium, akin to any Olympic platform, to receive and proudly wear the gold medal of survival and esteem.

I respect Callie for hanging in there. I know firsthand that she has endured great emotional pain. The intensity of that pain, of course, was a reflection of the degree of loss of potential with which she lived. The neglect and abuse that she suffered as she grew up left her unwittingly weakened. But she made it!

Only now does Callie have a future to which she can look forward. She sees herself in a job she likes—one in which she can achieve in ways she hadn't been able to earlier. And she wants to continue the networking she's been able to do with agencies and people in her community.

"I've sort of become an ADD magnet at the library. I'm very protective of the children who come to me. Some are sent by a local psychologist. I find myself reaching out to help ADD kids be who they are," she says. In fact, her job has worked out well for her in many ways. "I have a lot of flex time on my job. I like that. One thing that is good about it is that I can do a lot of things—work for a while in the morning, go to a meeting, work on a project, go out on the bookmobile, and then sit and prepare book orders. I love the variety.

"My supervisor values the things that I can do and is not a stickler for the things I struggle with. She's aware of ADD. And she gave me over $2,000 for ADD materials, and are they ever used!"

With a smile in her voice Callie says, "At fifty-five, I can honestly say I've never been happier in my entire life. I'm not in utopia, but I'm not constantly having to go back to work to finish, as I did when I was younger. The medication has been key for me, but not the whole thing!"

Then, almost poignantly, she adds, "I hope I can stay." (Just before the printing of this book Callie received a job commendation and pay increase.)

Each time I see or talk to Callie, I see the enormous strides she has taken. Not too long ago, I started to hear a shift in her voice—a calm, comfortable sound that literally brought tears to my eyes. And I wondered about that change.

Callie answers my silent question when she says, "I've slowed down. People need to do that either through meditation or whatever, so they can experience introspection. The key is to be kind to yourself while doing this. I've learned to do it. I look back and have compassion for myself instead of criticism.

"I see the future as kind of . . . happy," she says, and then adds, "Happy, maintaining the status quo." Music to my ears! Joy to her heart!

She continues, "My fantasy future would be to maintain my health, be active, and be able to physically function on twenty acres in a log cabin that has no electricity. That is a very physical thing for me."

What Works For and Against Callie

Sensitivity is absolutely the number one attribute shaping Callie's life. If ever anyone represented the misunderstood ADD child, Callie would be that person. A *hellion* and *mean* were terms applied to a child so sensitive that all she could do was try in the only way she knew to counteract the pressures of insensitivity and hurt that struck her.

The setup for her impulsive behavior started early with her mother's needs and her father's words. "If there had been a hospital room available, your mother would have aborted you," she remembers her father saying; the words registered deep within her psyche.

"I was in a lot of pain growing up. I felt very alone," she says. "Part of it was that pervasive feeling of having something wrong with me that I couldn't put my finger on. Consequently, I was very sensitive to other people who hurt. When they hurt, I felt it."

Now, that pain and sensitivity translate into empathy and compassion. When she was a child, they didn't. Then, when another child was hurting, it reminded her of her own pain, and she had to do something to stop the pain. So, when James—the neighborhood boy she and her friends treated so poorly—came around carrying his pain, she was the one who "acted out," trying to drive him out of her space.

It wasn't that she wasn't empathetic. She was too empathetic. She felt too much. Initially a liability, Callie's sensitivity has been transformed into a beautiful aspect of her adult personality.

Another ADD attribute that shows itself in many settings is Callie's ability to think from a variety of angles. "Sometimes people think I'm fence-sitting, "she says. "But I can see things from different perspectives. It helps me in my relationships with people. I don't have the concept that what I'm thinking is always right or the only right way."

Working as a professional librarian, Callie says she has difficulty with her ADD when she's "focusing and maintaining her attention through sequencing. I have to handle statistics off a computer sheet and put them on a kind of template that gets photocopied. I can repeat it (the handling of the statistics) monthly, but I have to go through dailies and put stats on this sheet. And I leave things out. It's one of those things I know that I do, so I try really, really hard to double-, even triple-check my figures. I'll think I did a wonderful job, and I'll go back the next day, and there will be holes in it. I will have gone through it, and I won't have completed a step."

Well, join the crowd, Callie! In response I say with a laugh, "If I had to do whatever you're talking about, I'd have been fired long ago." What Callie expects of herself is amazing. I never cease to wonder!

But she wants to be able to keep the data. She likes being a librarian even though that part of it is difficult for her. With medication it's possible, but still hard, for her to do all parts of her job well. To be sure, she feels frantic at times and frustrated at other times. But she also has come to realize she wants to do it. She realizes her brainwiring gets in the way. She's come to grips with the challenge she faces and no longer feels she's less valuable because of her difficulty with keeping statistics. Hurrah!

Callie now accepts the fact that often she really is wrong, not just feeling as if she is wrong. As she says, "I've covered so long that people don't realize I'm frequently actually wrong. Yes, I tend to be a pleaser, but I also know, now, that I'm truly error-prone, so I tend to accommodate by going over and over my work." However, she does not particularly see this as a liability—just as something with which she needs to work.

WHAT CALLIE WANTS YOU TO KNOW

You've got to know that there's another way to live.

Feel it.

Feel confident.

Feel satisfaction when you've been able to complete a task. Life really can be better.

You can like yourself.

You can do things you couldn't do before.

Develop introspection.

Be kind to yourself.

Be who you are. Find your niche.

Bubba Pratt

My biggest challenge was being labeled "educably retarded" when I was eight years old. BP

And has he ever met that challenge! LW

It takes only seconds for me to figure out why people like Bubba. I'd been told how nice he was by the people who referred me to him, "He's a really nice guy." "Bubba is the best." "He's real." Three different statements from three different people.

I immediately pick up on the warmth in his voice as we talk. Here is a man who is at peace with himself and is sufficiently secure to give to, as well as take from, others. I know automatically he won't be a hurtful person by being either critical or cold.

During our conversation, he tells me about something he'd read that beautifully explains the tone I was hearing. "Dogs that are the most secure never bite you," he says, "but the dogs that are the most insecure are most likely to bite."

Then he explains how he's arrived at the "nonbiting" place in his life. "I used to be that way. I used to bite people. It was called a temper. I was very insecure. People were continually putting me down. People were constantly telling me how dumb I was. So, if a person looked at me wrong, I started a fight," Bubba says. "As I started reading and becoming more secure with myself, I could be comfortable with who I am. I learned that who I am is okay, so I stopped biting. I know now it's okay for me to be how I am."

ADD functions constantly in Bubba's life, as it does for many of us in various degrees. Not only does it make him good at what he does, but it also causes him to farm out lots of jobs—and makes him have to apologize with considerable regularity.

"I miss a lot of appointments," he says. "I have to do a lot of calling and apologizing for missing them, and I have to do a lot of calling and apologizing for being late. It drives me crazy, but for some reason, I'm usually late."

His solution, however, also reflects his ADD problem-solving skills and wonderfully innocent honesty. "I think I'm transparent, and I go out and let people know what I'm like. I tell them I'm very disorganized. I tell them I have a challenge with this and please have patience with me and don't let this stand in our way."

He also surrounds himself with organized people who can help him. He continually works on self-improvement, and now that he knows about being ADD, Bubba focuses his attention on learning to accommodate his vulnerabilities.

Oh, yes, did I forget to mention it? Bubba is a millionaire. And his financial well-being is because his ADD attributes have provided him with the skills of sensitivity, empathy, people-intelligence, a vision of the big picture, and the willingness to take on challenges.

Bubba's Background

The middle child of three, Bubba was raised in Columbus, Georgia, where his father was a school principal and his mother a medical-office manager. He says, "I had a good family life. I had real good parents. My father was an encourager. He kept telling me that I was not dumb. My mother was outgoing and very supportive. She nurtured me a lot and believed in me. She was a typical protective mom."

Talking to an obviously articulate, intelligent man made me wonder why this issue of "dumbness" kept coming up. It didn't take long to get the rest of the story.

Bubba backs into it, saying, "I failed third grade. The school had me tested by a psychologist. Back in the sixties when a psychologist came in, that person would be the psychologist for the whole county." Chuckling, he adds, "Today, you've got a psychologist, a doctor, a nurse, a policeman, and three FBI agents in every school. Back in those days, the things that were considered bad were a kid speaking out of turn and chewing gum and sticking it under the desk. Those were major offenses."

In retrospect, I realize I'd gotten so caught up in his humorous storytelling that I'd forgotten the twang of pain I felt when he'd mentioned failing third grade. I'd even forgotten where we were headed in the interview, thanks to his skill as a communicator. And I failed to realize that probably Bubba, too, at least unwittingly, wanted to stay away from the pain of what he was going to tell me.

But Bubba gets back on track, saying, "Well, I'd failed the third grade and my father came to meet with the principal. The principal was a good friend of my father's. I sat outside the office while they talked. I was just sitting there like any kid, looking all over the place, a little bit nervous."

Can't you see the little boy in your mind, feet dangling, legs not long enough to place those feet on the floor, bored and hoping the time would pass quickly so he could get past his anxiety?

"I could hear the men talking and my dad asked, 'What's Bubba got?'

" 'Well, Ralph,' the principal said, 'Bubba's been diagnosed as being educably retarded.' "

In his inimitable adult fashion, Bubba says, "I didn't know

what 'educably' was, but I knew what 'retarded' was. I felt my heart go to my feet, my eyes welling up with tears, thinking, 'Oh God, I'm retarded.'

"It was the biggest blow I've ever had in my life.

"They found out I couldn't read at all. I couldn't even read the simplest book. So my dad put me in a reading center. Even by the time I got to college, I could only read at the sixth grade level.

"My dad kept telling me, 'You're not dumb. You're a very smart boy.' He just figured I had a reading problem. He didn't know about dyslexia, which is how I would be labeled now, but he didn't buy into the fact that I was retarded. He knew better than that. But he didn't know what it was."

With tears in my eyes and tightness in my chest, I comment to the adult Bubba, "Today, you are the product of his faith in the unknown."

"That's right," were the simple words that came back from him. But they were encased in the thankfulness and love of a grown son toward the father who probably saved his life. Bubba's father improved his son's self-esteem, so that later, healing of such a deep wound could occur. He's also the product of a mother and grandmother who read to him by the hour. He recalls sitting in a rocking chair by the fireplace watching the video created in his mind by hearing the stories. And Bubba learned.

Bubba is not retarded. Bubba would be classified as severely dyslexic and ADD, which he found out in 1995 when his daughter was diagnosed with dyslexia and attention deficit disorder.

Bubba says, "I was sitting with my daughter's counselor, who said, 'A lot of times this is hereditary.' I told her I didn't know what dyslexia was and I didn't know what ADD was, so she gave us a video to take home and my wife said, 'That's you. You have this. That's you.'

"I went back and was talking to the psychologist. She knew I was successful in the community and wondered how I'd

98

overcome my dyslexia and ADD and I said, 'It was easy because until five minutes ago I didn't know I had them.'"

Bubba's success at surviving came because his parents didn't quit believing in him. They gave him the most important ingredient of success: a successful attitude. His successful attitude shows when he talks about his daughter and her future. Bubba says, "Instantly, the thought that came to my mind when my daughter was diagnosed was, 'The toughest thing she's going to have to do is go through school, but that's the most insignificant thing she'll do in her life.'"

Bubba says his daughter's psychologist backed him up when she explained, "If we can just protect your daughter's self-esteem, then she will excel." And excelling is just what she is doing, with guidance, educated support, and people who believe in her—just like her grandparents believed in her dad.

But it has taken Bubba longer to get his life together than it will likely take his daughter. Reading classes didn't much help. He even set a goal during his freshman year in college to work on his reading that so he could achieve a ninth-grade level by the end of the year. But he never cracked a book.

How in the world did Bubba even get to college? His ticket was athletics. Back in second grade, his teacher, "a really nice lady," told his dad, "If I could just keep Bubba inside the class instead of fishing or playing football, then Bubba would do well." She said she just couldn't keep his attention inside the classroom.

Basically, most of his teachers liked him, and some probably sensed hidden intelligence that tests didn't reflect. His elementary school principal helped him get to middle school. His dad, the principal in middle school, helped him get to high school. And the principal in high school helped him get to college. And throughout everything, athletics helped him want to stay in school.

Frankly, if Bubba had been barred from athletics, I don't think his life would have turned out as well as it did. He played all sports through the early years and later concentrated on track and football.

How sad that the road to athletics must move through the academic classroom when two totally different sets of intelligences are involved. A person who is skilled in the verbal or mathematical areas does not have to prove himself in physical activity in order to get on with life and be called successful. The same is not true in reverse. Far too many children are discriminated against or told, "You could do your school work if you'd just try harder. You may not play sports or engage in extra-curricular activities for the next six weeks. Only if you pass everything, can you play after that." Punishment and threats do not help youth who don't fit the educational system. They only harm these youngsters.

The knowledge about learning differences is available, but it is not utilized. I often think what today's world would be like if the technology that runs our cars or computers was kept on the shelf because people believe you could get a horse to run faster if only it wanted to. We're losing a lot of human potential by ignoring different forms of learning styles.

With some understanding of the bleak picture I'm painting, Bubba's dad did what many parents find they have to do in order to save their children. He carried tests home from school so that Bubba could take them before he took the test in school. He did what he had to do for his kid. It's called survival.

Offered a football scholarship to many colleges across the country, Bubba started college at the University of Florida. He describes how the head coach walked in and told the academic coach, "Bubba's going to need a lot of pass/fail classes, easy ones."

"I never graduated," he said, "though I accumulated over 120 hours, finally declaring as a recreation major." In college, his most memorable experience academically was with a professor he describes as "an angel who dropped out of heaven."

Bubba says, "I couldn't take tests, especially multiple choice tests. I could never get past the questions even if I knew the answers. This professor said, 'You're a very intelligent person and you're a good person, and we're going to figure out what's wrong with you.'"

With a little stress in his voice even today, Bubba describes how the professor took him under his wing. For a young man whose father had died early—Bubba was only eighteen at that time—this professor must have felt like a godsend. What a gift!

"He worked with me with the test and basically did the same thing that my dad had done. Before I'd go take the test, I would sit in his office and study it. I'd come in early, and he'd give me the test orally. I'd pass the test. Then I'd go take the test, and I couldn't pass it writing it."

Fortunately, Bubba has an excellent memory. Once information is presented to him, he retains it. He remembers names well. He simply doesn't process written information particularly well, and he is also compromised in the expressive writing area. But using other means for obtaining information, especially hands-on teaching, a show-me-don't-tell-me approach, Bubba can use the wonderful intelligence with which he is gifted.

Today he knows this. Recently he bought a computer and had the same person who had taught his daughter how to use hers come and teach him to use his. The teacher read the manual and showed Bubba what to do. Bubba learned how to use his computer by being allowed to explore this new challenge on his own terms and experimenting with the computer directly.

Bubba married during his junior year in college. He laughs saying, "I married my opposite. Sandy is fun, my best friend, and very organized. She was a good student in high school and placed second highest in the school math contest. Here was this guy who can't add two and two, and Sandy's figuring out these equations."

Eighteen years later, they have five children, a great multilevel marketing business, and plenty of time to have fun and be philanthropic, which is what they like to do with their extra money. But such a good state of affairs was not always the case.

As a junior in college, Bubba wanted to play professional football. Coaches and sports experts predicted that he would be drafted within the first five rounds of the NFL football draft the following year, but it didn't happen the way he, or anyone, expected. A coaching change occurred and all the seniors were benched for the last four games of the season as the coaches were trying to work their new players. "So," Bubba says, "I didn't get drafted."

"What did you do?" I ask, feeling anxiety in my heart. Bubba responds, "An alumnus offered me a job selling shoes. I guess I was just a nice guy. I did that for four years. But I wasn't making it. I couldn't even pay the utility bill. My wife and I had our first baby when a previous football booster offered me a job selling cars.

"I tried it. I figured I had to do something. The first three months I likely starved to death. Then I changed again and went to another car dealership and got around the right people. They were really honest, ethical people, and I stayed seven years and did a good job.

"Then in 1985, I saw the particular multilevel marketing business I got into. Two other times I'd been exposed to it. The first time an explanation of it went right over my head—the guy was talking about business and how business works. Sandy was picking up on everything, but I wasn't. The second time I was exposed to it, I even tried one meeting but didn't make a sale. I quit.

"But in 1985 it was different. This time I was looking at a representative of the business, not the business." Someone befriended him, explained the business to him, and took an interest in Bubba, the person. Listening to him, I thought, how ADD it was to be able to distinguish between a people-oriented meeting and a "thing"-oriented meeting.

As if he were reading my mind, Bubba says, "It's like going into a restaurant, and you have a bad waiter or waitress and you walk out and you say, 'I'm never going to get in that section again,' or you say, 'I'm not ever going to eat in that restaurant again.'" Just to be sure I get the analogy, he continues, "It's like not liking a book and saying, 'I'm not going to ever read another book.' I'd never met a good representative of the multilevel marketing business before."

Not only does Bubba respond to people better than to things, but by the time the third opportunity came around, he had five years of post-college living under his belt. He'd been learning in the environment in which he learns best—real life. And he was "needy," or at least he says he was.

Bubba puts it this way, "I asked the guy to look me in the eye and tell me, 'You can do this.' Well, he looked me in the eye all right and said, 'You can change,' meaning he was looking at a twenty-eight-year-old guy living in an eleven-hundred-square-foot house, who couldn't pay his mortgage, couldn't pay his car payment, and never balanced a checkbook. I was just a wreck financially."

Bubba continues somewhat muted in his tone. "Then he looked directly at me. I had on a brown and beige penguin shirt with two buttons and a red and gray tie that was tied by my father in 1977 when my neck was twenty-two and a half inches. That tie remained tied from 1977 until 1985, when my post-football neck was only seventeen inches. The big part came up to my chest and the little part came down to my stomach. This is what the guy was looking at. I was not the model of success."

Years later, Bubba asked that man what he had seen in him. The man answered, "I saw a hard worker, a person who was a good person, and a person who wanted to provide for his family."

"Basically what he told me was that if I wanted to become successful, I'd need to know there's a reason why you are the way you are—usually, it's because of what you've learned, what you've done in the past. And if you want to change, you change what you're doing," Bubba says.

Bubba decided he needed to become educated and took to heart the advice of those who were willing to help him. He began to memorize words. Fortunately that assignment was one that he could master with the style of brainwiring he has. He also memorized Bible verses. And he started to read fifteen minutes a day even though he only read two pages at first.

His study program, his wife Sandy's help in the business, and his mentor's guidance led him to add $2,000 per month to his income in the first year. Now he makes a seven-figure income annually.

But making money isn't the only payoff, though initially it was his first and foremost goal. "I look at money like it is a tool. If you're unhappy without it, you'll be miserable with it. Happiness is an inside job. Now I help people with scholarships, I mentor kids, I coach junior high football and I use money in a lot of different ways—all to help people."

When I First Met Bubba

Initially I came to know Bubba through others who have worked with him, and I heard the same story over and over. One of Bubba's college coaches said it well: "Here's Bubba Pratt, number 60 on the field and number one in your heart."

This guy has that wonderful charm that is often associated with ADD. There's more to Bubba than that, though. "At first," he says, "I'm shy until I get to know you." A lot of us made this way "flood" (become overwhelmed) easily in new situations. It takes a little time to figure out what's going on and what's expected. All the stimuli that others may ignore, we take in. He says, "Until I can get it organized, I stay quiet. Being quiet keeps me from making mistakes and putting my foot in my mouth."

But he also is very, very sensitive, like a lot of people who have

ADD wiring. That sensitivity has led to lots of hurt along the way for him. Not the usual "bullshit artist," someone afraid to feel feelings, Bubba shows real courage in owning his feelings.

He relates an example of his sensitivity in response to my question about his intuition. "I can sense things," he says. "I can tell when someone agrees or disagrees, and I can tell when I've hit a real touchy area. I can feel what people are feeling. For example, if a person passes away, I can feel the spouse's pain. I'm very empathic."

Then he adds, "It's just amazing. I'm not an emotional person, but when someone has pain, I get real emotional. It's the weirdest thing—I can literally feel what they feel."

How Bubba Envisions the Future

Speaking of feeling emotional, Bubba says, "I see the future as bright and big because no matter what happens, I can make it bright and big. I realize everything I have now can be gone. To be honest I couldn't give a rip. I don't care, because what I have doesn't make me happy. It's what I've become. I look at losses like adversity. Adversity is preparation. It prepares me for something great down the road."

It seems to me that Bubba has become a lot like the way he describes his dad. "I think he was wise," says Bubba. "He had a master's degree from Auburn, but he was just wise. He could think on his feet. One day someone could say something like, 'I'm tired of this crap,' and instead of him reacting, he'd just say something with a smile and you'd just have to laugh."

Bubba plans to continue to use his resources and past experience to serve as a model for others—especially youth who otherwise wouldn't have a chance of succeeding. The first thing he tells the freshman junior varsity team he coaches is that he, too, was in special education classes.

There's no comeback to Bubba's honesty, even for a kid who is ashamed or feeling sorry for himself because he's not as bright as the next guy or as talented or whatever. He shares, "When they say, 'Hey coach, you don't understand, I'm this and I'm dumb,' I start talking to them about special education. Their eyes get big, and they ask me how come I know so much about special education.

"I tell them. 'I was in special education.' Then I do things with them. I help put them in career programs. I give them books and work with them and talk with them and let them know there is a bright side and that what they do now is important. I tell them, 'The people who discourage you, you can't listen to them. The people who encourage you, gravitate toward them.'

"And I tell them, 'Let me tell you what one of my teachers told my wife's mother. She said that she couldn't believe that my wife was marrying some idiot like me whose fist was bigger than his brain and the marriage wouldn't last two years. Other teachers said I needed to go out and get a job where I would use my arms and back, because that's the only thing that I had in my body that was strong.'"

Then with pride in his voice, he shows the kids his car—a Mercedes Benz. He's not bragging about what he has, but is joyful for a bunch of kids who know the value of his car. He knows how to reach them. He knows what's important to them.

In response he hears, "Wow! Bubba," as they begin to realize that perhaps they, too, can make it.

Bubba wants to keep on giving to young people. When I ask him about what kids need to get from him, he hesitates, thinking. After a pause, he says, "I think the biggest thing . . . I'd try to convince a young person . . ." That's as far as Bubba gets.

Then I realize what is happening. This strong, successful man is tearing up. I sense that he is revisiting some of the pain he lived through as a youth, when he didn't have the knowledge and understanding that he has today. I wait.

Resuming with a soft but clear voice, he says, "I'll try to convince a kid that no matter what anybody says, that he just needs to believe in himself and realize he can overcome anything that's out there that he has to face. Time is on his side."

It is my turn to choke up. And I do. Don't those of us who have struggled with ADD feel those same feelings from our own youth? Don't we care for those who follow in the ensuing generations? And don't we want them to be spared the pain of criticism, feelings of inadequacy, and impoverished self-worth?

What Works For and Against Bubba

Bubba has a bunch of ADD characteristics that work for him. But because he has barely gotten used to the idea that he is constructed in the ADD way, he doesn't really associate many of his strongest assets with ADD. Nevertheless, he is what he is in large part because of ADD traits that work for him.

He's been able to use these traits even when the odds were stacked against him as a child. His parents and mentors gave him the gifts that make the difference. They didn't feel sorry for him or allow him to become helpless and "handicapped." Instead they believed in him, so he could believe in himself. They shielded him from undue pressures and expectations until he grew strong enough to defend himself and learn the skills of negotiation, so that he could trade in the best interest of all the parties involved.

More than once Bubba says, "I was lucky." He knows that athletics in the early years was his saving grace. As he puts it, "I had nothing else to help my self-esteem. So I was fortunate to have that special talent. It helped me succeed."

What Bubba learned in athletics he continues to use: sportsmanship, spontaneity, leadership, and teamwork. With a high level of interpersonal intelligence, Bubba has teamed with his wife Sandy to make a go of a business that can use his people skills to advantage.

He uses his ADD creativity to advantage but not as one might expect. He solves people-problems creatively. He counsels people. He says, "I sit down with someone and I help them. For example, I had a person come up to me one time, and he said, 'I have serious marital problems.' I said, 'I know.' And he said, 'Oh, my gosh, I can't believe it. Is it that obvious? How did you know?'

"And I answered him, 'You're married.' He laughed, we sat down and we talked. He said, 'What should I do?' I told him, 'I think you should write a list of things you would like your wife to do, kinds of attitudes you would like her to have, what you'd like her to cook for breakfast for you. Write a list of everything you'd like your wife to do and be.' He wrote the list and asked, 'Are you going to go talk to her?'

"I said, 'No, you're going to work to become that person. You become that kind of person, and then she'll become that kind of person.'"

My immediate thought upon hearing his story is that his advice happens to be brilliant. I tell him. Then it occurs to me that perhaps Bubba doesn't see himself as brilliant, so I ask, "You know that, don't you?"

"No, I don't know that," he replies.

Instantly, I realize that he hadn't learned the technique cognitively. He hadn't read any theories of marriage counseling in a book. He just knew. And sure enough, he continues, "Those are just things—I don't know how I do it. I don't know where it comes from, but I sit down, and I can help people with things like that."

Not only does Bubba get an A+ in marriage counseling, but, thanks to his ADD traits, he has really made a difference in that man's life.

Bubba helps others be honest with themselves and he practices what he preaches. Whether working with his wife or sharing about his ADD attributes, Bubba says, "I am transparent." That is, he lets people see him inside and out, the whole Bubba, not a social mask or a package of "well-socialized" behaviors. "I didn't always do that," he says. "I had to learn to be open. I just started doing it."

Yes, Bubba practices what he preaches. He communicates with his wife a lot. They have been a team for a long time and he plays straight with his partner, Sandy. With his permission and desire, he lets her bug him when things need to get done.

"She sits over me and says, 'You've got to do this. You've got to do this.' And I do it." Bubba listens. The work gets done and no one is the worse off because of the way in which they accomplish what needs to be done. Each has a job. Each respects the other's skills. And each contributes to a team approach that has brought them success. Without Bubba's ADD attributes, they wouldn't be so successful.

They've even learned as partners to deal with a somewhat disconcerting ADD attribute, the "uh-huh" phenomenon. Let's say Sandy asks Bubba a question. Because his attention is elsewhere, he says, "Uh-huh," having heard that a question was asked but not really processing what the question was.

Bubba instantly gives me a great example. "Like when I was going up to Canada, my wife said, 'Do you have the boys' passports?' I said, 'Uh-huh.' At that she just got up, went to the safe, got the boys' passports out, and put them in my calendar book."

Apparently his "uh-huh" didn't put Sandy off track into assuming that he'd completed the task. No doubt from experience, she knew what his "uh-huh" meant. Neither did she feel put out or annoyed. That means she, too, has achieved peace with certain ADD attributes of her mate.

He does, however, still struggle with the afterimage of his previous self-esteem issues. Bubba succinctly explains, "Until recently, I didn't know I was ADD, so I've had to get life right in spite of it. I had no one working with me. I had to do what I had to do. I couldn't sit down. I couldn't study longer than ten minutes. It frustrated me how people could study for two hours. I'd study and then go out in the hall and do stupid stuff like shoot my bow and arrow at the garbage can—I'm still like a durn kid."

At that, I confront Bubba, asking, "Why do you label what you did 'stupid?'"

"I'm trying to get out of that habit, but I think it's something that people have laid on me all my life. So I kind of bought into it as a defense mechanism, like when they said, 'You're retarded.' I remember sitting outside that principal's office going, '*Urrrrr, urrrr,*' running my finger quickly back and forth across my lips so I made a vibrating sound. You know, the kind that means 'stupid.' I either cried or did that."

For Bubba, an identification of ADD and dyslexia has been liberating. He never was "stupid" or "retarded." But he's still dealing with the shame and pain of his initial labeling. He must leave the idea behind that there is something wrong with him. He will in time.

WHAT BUBBA WANTS YOU TO KNOW

Believe in yourself.

You have abilities and talents.

Failure is temporary.

Never give up trying.

Every situation presents an opportunity.

Have the right attitude.

There's something great waiting for you.

Boo Capers

We're not here to be miserable.   BC

And Boo shows us how to have fun.   LW

Eyes wide as saucers, face round as a plate, Boo Capers is impossible to overlook. Her energy is big. Her voice is full. Her stature is impressive. Her talent is expansive. Her charisma automatically draws others to her—and, by reports, it's been that way since she was a tiny tot.

The results of Boo's active imagination often got her into trouble, like the day in fifth grade when she went to school with a plaster cast on her arm so that she wouldn't have to take a test for which she'd failed to study. Not only was she excused from taking the test, but she received a lot of attention for her broken arm.

Everything was going along according to plan until her arm felt hot and the cast felt scratchy. What did Boo do? The practical thing, of course. She went to the girls' restroom and took off her cast.

Her family's response: "She's just being Boo!"

Neither Boo nor her family knew about ADD when she was growing up. As an adult, she became a school teacher and was aware that she had kids in her classroom labeled ADD. But Boo saw them as creative, unique, and full of energy and fun. She realized then that she was the same way. Boo is still "just being Boo" as she approaches the fifth decade of her life. Throughout her life, she has consistently retained a sense of humor, creativity, and an adventurous spirit.

Somewhere between her creative/expressive genius and being a free spirit who values her freedom more than anything else in life, Boo makes her living dreaming up fantasy programs for the children she teaches in Dallas, Texas. Working mostly with young children, she contracts with schools to give children experiences in creative dramatics. In addition she runs after-school and summer programs at her studio school, to which children flock to have fun with theater and art experiences.

As she says, "I can stay a child at my creative drama school. I love it."

Of all the people I know, Boo has probably changed the least in the eighteen years I've known her. She has kept the joyful exuberance of a young person. Her energy remains high and she continually enjoys new creative challenges. I never know what creative project she'll come up with next. And from family reports, we can tack on another thirty years of consistent expression at being who she is, has been, and may well always be.

Boo's Background

The youngest of three children, Boo has a sister and brother eight and six years older, respectively. Seeing her sister Nancy in a motherly light, Boo followed her everywhere.

Boo tells me, "I liked to do everything." Usually when I hear this, I figure the person is simply not aware of how they spend their time. But with Boo, the statement is nearly true. "Just being Boo," also meant getting into lots and lots of things, in the house and out.

When pressed, she tells me that she loved to play dress-up, put on patio shows, and organize plays, all precursors to her career in creative drama. In addition, she loved creating music, singing, and making people laugh. Then there were the outdoor activities such as building environments—could this be a predecessor to designing and building theater sets?—building forts, and playing in creeks and neighborhood drain pipes.

Lots of time was spent playing games with others—her sister, brother, and neighborhood friends, including "Boing-Boing," her running buddy. Would you like to take a guess about how "Boing-Boing" is wired? In fact, if I could find him, I might want to include him in this book.

As a child, Boo had a tremendous amount of natural curiosity and she struggled with boredom. She slowly became aware that she could do well in school if she wanted to. "If I was interested in the class or liked the teacher, I did fine. But I wouldn't pay attention when I got bored."

That combination—natural curiosity and struggle with boredom—led to some interesting escapades, such as the time in second grade when she had collected little metal disks—the kind used in electrical sockets. She found them while exploring houses that were being built near her home. She knew she wasn't supposed to be in the houses, but, as she says, "I never did like rules very much." Then she adds, "I was never bad. I mostly just got bored, so I got in trouble."

When show-and-tell time was announced at school, she bagged up her metal disks and took them for her presentation. There was only one other little girl in class with her. All the rest of her classmates were boys—to whom she related better than to the girls.

When the girl asked, "What's in the bag? Candy?" Boo wouldn't tell her. The girl kept "bugging" Boo. Irritated at the whiny pressure, Boo opened the bag and gave her some disks, saying, "You can't taste it until you swallow it."

The disks had sharp edges. The child swallowed one and was

rushed to the hospital. The disk was removed, and the child was fine.

Boo's seven-year-old response was, "Well, if she was dumb enough to eat it . . ."

Boo's parents didn't think much of their daughter's explanation. They responded immediately, explaining the danger of what she'd done. She definitely got the message never to do anything like that again.

It's a wonder, with Boo's cleverness and high level of creativity, that she didn't get into more trouble than she did. But what probably kept Boo on the straight and narrow were parents who were good models for appropriate behavior. Her parents both knew how to have fun themselves and how to be very serious with anything dangerous or potentially hurtful.

When her family said, "She's just being Boo," that didn't mean Boo was allowed to hurt others. It did mean that she was taught right from wrong and was loved and accepted for who she was, even though she sometimes did things that were not acceptable. Those lessons have stayed with her throughout her life, so that she has not had to struggle with feeling bad about herself as she's learned to control her curiosity and exuberance.

Boo was surrounded by people when she was little, she says, and rarely had time to be alone. In adulthood, she has managed to keep a balance between being gregarious and solitary. But she loves her time alone after the high-level social activities she enjoys through her profession. She uses her time off in her garden or in projects such as learning to master video production, and spends hours of solitary time editing to achieve the results she desires.

Fly-fishing, though, is Boo's all-time favorite avocation—she's absolutely enamored with this sport and has been for five years. She describes the experience as being immersed in the elements and sharing the environment with its natural inhabitants.

It's hard to believe that Boo was sick as a child, starting out as a blue baby who had lots of problems with her lungs. Nevertheless, she says, "what I remember most is having fun. Life was fun. My mother, sister, and brother are all hyper. My father was a wonderful storyteller and an eloquent wordsmith. I miss him since he died in 1989."

When you listen to Boo talk about herself as a child and watch the expressions on her face, you know that she hasn't created a fantasy childhood. In fact, she apparently lived in an entertainment center, with lots of freedom to be herself. She was able to express herself openly and funnel happiness to and from those around her. This same attitude of enjoyment pervades Boo's creative-drama school and her relationships with the children she teaches.

It's no wonder that she went into the entertainment business when she grew up. "I always liked kids," she says, and she became involved in children's theater in high school. "I wanted to be a singer and wanted to work with children and music. I tried playing in clubs for a number of years but that got old real fast, and eventually I concentrated on teaching children. They're a lot more fun than grown-ups, who have a lot of trouble letting down so they can be expressive. It's hard to work with adults. They're so stiff that I have to spend all my time breaking through their inhibitions. With children I can get to the expressive part right away. I don't have the patience to spend a lot of time getting ready to be expressive."

Is Boo a Peter Pan, never having grown up? I don't think so. Naturally active and expressive, she has been given permission her whole life to honor that way of being. Rather than being saddled with oversocialization like so many of us, she has retained the freedom to be natural. This is her legacy to us.

Boo has a serious side that is incredibly sensitive and empathetic—so much so that she doesn't allow herself to linger long in the pain of worry and seriousness. When her school building was hit by a tornado a couple of years ago, sets were wrecked, long cherished costumes ruined, and her stage became unsafe for children to use. Most threatening and potentially expensive to fix, the building's roof was in question. Boo tells how she walked around in shock for a day, worrying about what she would do. She didn't know what her insurance would cover and how long it would take to fix things so that she could reopen for business. How was she going to make her living with no safe place for her to teach children?

One day was enough, though for Boo to mope around. The second day she went to work calling friends, relatives, parents of her students, anyone she could find to begin the massive repair job. And she worked fourteen- and sixteen-hour days to repair what had been destroyed. One month later to the day, Boo reopened her school. Enough insurance money was forthcoming to fix the roof and, with careful budgeting, even to make some improvements she'd been wanting to make before the storm.

She acknowledges the reality around her and then says, "Okay. That's enough. Time to move on." That's Boo. "I have big power" is how Boo describes her energy. And I promise you that is true. You always know when hearty-voiced Boo has moved into your space. She used to worry about her power, but not any more. As she says, "I've never allowed my power to get out of control." That's also true, undoubtedly in part because it's balanced with a high level of sensitivity and responsibility to others and her environment.

She has a heart that is easily hurt and realizes that others do, too. This has apparently heightened Boo's sensitivity to others—she knows what it's like to get hurt and doesn't want to impose it on anyone else. She reflects ADD sensitivity operating at its best.

When relationships aren't working, for example, Boo knows it's time to consider letting go of the friendship. First she sees whether the other person is available to work on fixing the problems between them. If not, she does her moving without leaving a mess behind. Boo also doesn't blame the other person or wallow around feeling guilty. She realizes they are both hurting and says so. Then it's time to let go cleanly.

I've often watched Boo with children. I've never seen her raise her voice or act angry. But I have seen her remain in control of situations that would bring others to their knees. Boo can manage a roomful of kids, move them from one area to another, and get them to do almost anything she wants, using the combination of her power and her sensitivity.

Children know what adults are feelings on the inside. They sense the adult's inner truth. And Boo's truth is kindness and firmness. She is not afraid of what children might do or say. She doesn't worry about their getting out of control. But then, she's not afraid of getting out of control herself. Combine that with the fact that she really likes children and likes herself, and you've got a workable combination that creates an environment in which children thrive.

When I First Met Boo

"Today, Boo showed us how the lights in the school auditorium work," said my older son, then eight. His brother, aged six, chimed in, "And she let me get on the stage and be a pumpkin. It was fun."

School hadn't been open for more than a few weeks when I was given daily reports, "Boo did this," and "Boo said that," and "Boo let us do this today." Considering that, like most parents, I was rarely given information about school even when I asked— much less voluntarily—I began to wonder who this Boo person was. And I wondered about her strange name.

So as a dutiful mother, I left work early one day to visit my sons' elementary school. Informed that Boo was in the auditorium, I made my way to the doors at the back and quietly and discreetly slipped in to observe what was going on.

I saw this energetic, vocal woman directing children around the stage. They were doing everything she asked and seemed to be having a lot of fun. She seemed to be taking equal pleasure in what they were doing. I quickly surmised that she liked her work.

I watched her manage even my own as-yet-unidentified ADD son, who was a bundle of joyful hyperactivity in motion. His exuberance was apparent, but he wasn't out of control even with a lot of activity going on around him. He seemed to gain control around Boo.

As the last of the children left, she made her way toward the back where I stood. I didn't know then, but I now know, that Boo doesn't miss anything. She'd noticed me the instant I came into the auditorium. But she also didn't miss a beat with what she was doing, figuring, I guess, that the kids were her first priority, and that I'd wait and probably not cause any trouble.

I soon understood why the kids talked so much about Boo. Her charisma wooed the children and helped them to express their creativity. They felt good about themselves and, in turn, felt good about her. Even my older son, who was not drawn to performance, was accepted and respected as he was. She put him in charge of lighting, a job he could do and one with which he felt comfortable. No child was pushed against his will or better judgment to do anything that didn't fit. He might be gently encouraged but was never pushed or shamed or forced. That was, and is, the magic of Boo.

In fact, she provided one of the few good school experiences for my younger ADD son up to that point. What I didn't realize at the time was the reason she could give him such empathy and good experiences: she used her own ADD sensitivity and empathy to provide what he and other children needed in order to feel good. After all, aren't some of our best teachers those who are ADD?

Over the years, Boo and I have become friends. Even though we often don't see each other for long periods of time, we're the kind of friends who can pick right up where we left off. She has continued to keep track of my children even though she no longer has any formal connection to them. And to this day, they smile when the name Boo is mentioned.

Boo gave me my one and only voice lesson. With no training or background, I had been hired to be a radio talk-show host. I called Boo to see if she would help me with my delivery on the air. At her studio she listened to me chatter as if I were on the air. Her only words were, "Talk more softly. Let the microphone do the work for you." I followed her advice and immediately became a hit, recognized and remembered because the tone quality of my voice helped people with their feelings. Listeners thought I'd had a lot of voice training, but I had one lesson with Boo. That's how effective she is as a teacher.

How Boo Envisions the Future

"I am looking forward right now to moving my school. I just signed a five-year lease on new space because I continue to feel strongly that children need to learn to understand their own experiences. And I need a new space to make sure I can work effectively with them. I want to continue to affirm and teach children. Each child is special to me. I honor each one. Each child is unique and wonderful.

"When people honor individuality, we discover that our strength lies in our differences. I say that every chance I get. I've spent eighteen years supporting diversity and still want to, enough that I've taken out that lease," Boo says.

And so Boo's future plans are likely to benefit a lot of young people. They will help make the world a better place in which to live. Boo continues to remind us, "We are not on this earth to be miserable, we are here to have fun!"

What Works For and Against Boo

Boo is strongly ADD and has many ADD attributes. But she does not suffer from them. Neither does she particularly accommodate them. She simply places herself in situations that reflect her assets positively and teams with others who have the skills she lacks.

Boo has been blessed to have been given permission to be who she is, naturally. Because of that, she has developed a lifestyle and career path that reflect her ADD attributes, using them to advantage. Everything that makes Boo a success in the world and within herself comes from these traits. She uses the gifts and talents with which she is endowed. She works on behalf of children, enriching their lives. And she brings creative, expressive enthusiasm into the lives of all those she touches.

Boo has beaten the odds and ignored the voices that tell people in this culture, "You can't make a good living being creative." She has systematically marched to her own drum. She is honest and forthright, following her dreams. And she has empowered thousands of others to do that, also.

Now teaching a second generation of children, she is being affirmed for the path she's chosen to follow. True, Boo was raised with an attitude that helped her achieve this perspective, but she has been the one to carry it further responsibly —passing it on to others.

My own ADD son, remarkably influenced by Boo, is now pursuing a teaching degree so that in his area of interest, sports, he can influence kids the way Boo does. I wonder to whom he will pass the baton. The lead runner will be remembered as a creative drama teacher who made a difference.

Boo's way of stating this synchronous state of affairs is, "I'm doing what God wants me to do. In the world, I'm in sync with who I am. I believe I'm a vehicle for God. I experience God as loving and I have feelings of love. I feel passionately about what I do. And I bring the same feeling out in children, parents, and everyone involved in the process."

Her organizational strengths show when she is designing something new, like the interior space of the building into which she is preparing to move. "I become intense at times like this," she says. "I see the vision, I walk through the school in my mind, and I love to put all this on paper. Getting ready is what I like, what I love.

"I enjoy the process—and I see life as a process, so things never end. I don't try to reach a goal. I just get started on something, and it goes on as long as I want it to and it never ends. I never experience finality. I stay in the process."

Boo has found one secret to mastering organization the ADD way. She brings a perspective to bear that escapes many people working with ADD. Usually, people with ADD traits have organizational problems when they try to deal with pieces of paper and data that don't interest them, do something that's not creative, or try to reach a goal that is of no importance to them.

Staying in the creative process means she honors the analog way of organizing that fits people who are ADD. In this sense, Boo has a perfectly good organizational system. She's figured out how to use her ADD for organizing rather than succumbing to the usual ADD organizational problems.

When it comes to keeping track of accounts for IRS purposes or doing bank statements and scheduling (linear organizational tasks), she hires someone who processes information differently than she does. She then gives them the freedom to do what they do well. Boo uses her ADD organization beautifully and respects others' ability to do what she doesn't want to do. And she doesn't press them to do the kind of creative development that she loves and does well.

Because of the way Boo looks at life and ADD, her ADD works for her and not against her. That's her secret.

Because of the way Boo looks at herself, I had to ask her a direct question to elicit any problems associated with her being ADD. I ask, "Have you ever had feelings of inadequacy that bother you?"

In response, she says, "There are things I couldn't understand in school, such as algebra. But I figured that just wasn't something that I was supposed to be able to know. I need things to be physical and sensible. I've known that for a long time. I do much better when I'm dealing with a practical situation. Algebra isn't practical."

She continues, "I'm not a quick study. I've had to work hard at school or to learn a lot of things. But I submerge myself in these things and accomplish what I want to if I'm interested.

"Because I have to work so hard, I have had feelings of inadequacy. So what I focus on is the process of doing things, not the end goal. That fits me better. And I don't feel inadequate as a result."

WHAT BOO WANTS YOU TO KNOW

Be honest and act ethically.

You have to believe in something. You've "gotta" do what feels good.

Trust your instincts.

Remember, you're not in control—God is.

Debbie Sager

Find what makes your light burn and others' warmth
will follow. DS

And she knows how to turn that light up. LW

Try following Debbie around for a few minutes, much less an hour, and you'll find out what it's like to ride on a roller coaster in the middle of a carnival. It's fun, educational, and never boring. Perhaps best of all, her whimsical, broad smile and twinkling eyes portray that she's enjoying herself, too. Well socialized, Debbie frowns a little, conveying the discomfort she feels by the expression on her face, which shows all. "I have a hard time focusing on one thing at a time in order to get through to the end without stopping and starting other things along the way," she says.

An example quickly follows without my having to prod her. "Just yesterday I was on my way to a going-away gathering for a neighbor of mine. I wanted to take a present but didn't want to spend much, so I quickly decided to make a birdhouse for her new yard."

The materials for the birdhouse were on Debbie's back porch, which also serves as the collection point for most everything that is on its way from her car, the surrounding woods, or anywhere else Debbie has been. Extricating the tools and materials needed to build the house from everything else that lay there was no mean feat.

A bit sheepishly Debbie murmured, "Building the birdhouse gave me the opportunity to sort through some things. I'd been thinking about wanting to put some of them away for a long time. So it seemed like the perfect opportunity. I realize in retrospect that it wasn't the time, but I was in the right space to do it, so I did. Then she added, chagrined, "I wasn't very late. I used to manage to suppress this kind of behavior, but now I prefer to be that way."

Debbie has two sides—the well-trained, socially aware, good-little-girl side and the highly expressive, creative, fun-loving-woman side. Her energy and joyfulness belie the number of years she's managed to accumulate. Sometimes when I'm around Debbie, I think of her as a bouncy sixteen-year-old. Rarely do I experience her as older than twenty-five—except for one reason. She's wise, way beyond her years.

Debbie talked about how she managed to conceal, even to herself, the ADD tendency to skip around and "get off track." "When I was in school, I simply didn't allow myself to do anything else besides the assignment of the moment—no diversions of any kind. When I needed a break I would do something directly related to the topic that I was supposed to be focusing on."

"If I needed to do math in college, I'd only let myself deal with things that were math related. When I needed to take a break, I'd divert myself by going through my checkbook—I'd allow myself to do only that. But I would be doing something related to the math homework because if I took a total break from it, I'd have a hard time getting back to it."

"I lived at home during part of college. My brother was multiply handicapped, so I lived in a special education family. When I needed a break from studying, I'd relate to my family, read a story about a special-ed person, or try out a theory at the state school—on-the-job training, you know. That was the only way I could keep focused on my special education studies."

Becoming more serious, Debbie tucked in her chin and sat a little straighter as she noted, "People say, 'Leave the office at home and do something different.' I am not able to do that because I can't bring myself back to the topic."

The twinkle returned to her eye and her voice became lyrical and playful as she said, "I'm fortunate, though, because now I'm teaching early childhood education, which is playful. I'm surrounded by toys and the time to play. And when I take a break, I play with different toys and watch kid's movies and TV shows and do things that are fun, including my arts and crafts—all things that are related to the topic."

As Debbie talked, I saw another aspect of her, one that I'd not seen before. It was almost as if she were getting away with something and was pleased at the idea. I could imagine a young child who pulled one over on her parents and was quite satisfied with herself as a result.

Debbie's Background

Just turning forty, Debbie has been a certified teacher for fifteen years, though she'll tell you that she began working at her profession when she was four. She is the older of two children by four years. Her brother James was healthy at birth, but all of that changed when he received his six-month pertussis vaccination and suffered an allergic reaction. His fever skyrocketed, causing seizures that cut off the blood flow from his brain for three minutes. He came out of the episode mentally retarded and epileptic, among other health problems.

That changed everything for Debbie and her family. As she says, "Instead of spending time on the playground, I was in neurologists' offices. I was learning about those things while other children were off on vacations. My family tried every magic cure there was, and I was a part of all of it."

Debbie retains a clear memory of her growing-up years in a small town in Central Texas. A handicapped brother, a mother, and a father made up her tiny world. Her dad took on the role of breadwinner, while her mother's job was to make sure the family was okay.

"This was a good separation of power that fit them," Debbie commented. "My dad was a man of action who had a compassionate side. But he'd been raised in a highly structured environment where there was only one *right* way to do things."

"His adult life was shaped by illness in two ways. His career in the navy, which he loved, was brought to an abrupt end when his mother became sick, and he felt he had to come back home. Instead of traveling the seas, he got a job at the local cotton mill, married my mother, and had us."

Ten years later, Debbie's dad's life was shaped by the catastrophic turn of events when his second child became ill. Again, his compassionate, responsible nature took over, directing him to stay at the mill where he had insurance for his son, who was not insurable elsewhere.

So Debbie's father's desire for action was curtailed somewhat. He did, however, work as a maintenance supervisor and electrician so he was able to move around. Debbie, sympathizing with her father, said, "He got to do a variety of things, but he never got the freedom that an action person would like."

Debbie figures that her dad would probably have gone into business for himself if her brother hadn't become ill. "He was a very good electrician. He could fix anything. He would have loved the freedom of having his own business and would have done well because he was so conscientious." At that she sighed the sigh of an understanding daughter who wished her father could have more nearly approximated his potential before he died in 1988.

I came to understand that some of the wisdom and compassion Debbie communicates comes from the experiences of living in her family and some from her own innate sensitivity to others. She confided, "I was taught growing up that people were the most important thing—they come first. You could have a messy house. You could go without food. You could have other problems, but as long as people were taken care of, that was most important. And that's my natural inclination anyway."

Debbie and her dad, both sensitive and attuned to feelings, did not have an exclusive edge on feelings. "My Mom," Debbie continued, "is a *very* feelings-type person. She and I are a lot alike in that respect. But in contrast to me, she also likes a lot of organization. She likes to fit things into their little slots."

Thoughtfully, she added, "She's more methodical than I remember. Some of the things she did, I now realize she did because they were good for my brother, but I think she's more structured than I thought."

Continuing to ponder, Debbie noted, "I talk about her as if I'm away from her. And I have been. She and my brother had a real symbiotic relationship. When my brother died in 1986, I had to get to know my mother all over again. I found the mother I lost at four. She came back. She had to find herself, too."

Debbie's dad, inventive, restless, creative as he was, probably supplied some of Debbie's ADD genes. Because of the way he was raised, he was able to inhibit a lot of his natural tendency toward activity. Highly responsible, he kept a tight rein on his emotions and his behavior.

Debbie's mother, too, demonstrates some ADD traits. Emotionally sensitive, she feels things deeply, picks up minute cues from others, and lives through her feelings. This level of sensitivity is characteristic of all forms of ADD, including Highly Structured ADD (see introduction); her need and desire for structure and compartmentalization are traits of this third type of ADD and probably reflect the predominant form of her ADD attributes. Unable to change gears readily, people with this form of ADD cannot easily switch tracks and do not like flexible situations. They automatically tend to work within a structure because it feels good to them.

Debbie is a combination of both parents. More like her father, she is active, restless, inventive, and very creative as well as highly sensitive. Though she doesn't appear naturally to have the Highly Structured ADD traits of her mother, she tried, when she was younger, to emulate them for survival purposes. Her father's training as a highly responsible person also rubbed off on her.

The result makes Debbie a study in contrasts—a fun-loving, bubbly woman who catastrophizes situations. Mixing the highly structured learning she received with the empathetic, sensitive nature of a dramatic personality, you get a tendency to expect the worst. She says, "When I think of the worst possible scenario, I can prepare myself to meet it."

For example, when a torrential rainstorm hit the Austin, Texas, area recently, she said, "I began to worry because my son had gone to a movie with a neighbor, and I just knew they'd be caught in the storm. In my mind I could see the car skidding off the road, rolling over, and everyone in it being hurt. I could hear my son calling, 'Help me.'"

She continued, "By the time they got home, I had already figured out whom I would call to help me and what I would do about my job while I nursed my son back to health. What a relief to see him fine and in one piece!"

Dramatic? Yes. Mentally creative? Yes. Mentally unstable? No. Debbie knows even as she is worrying that she is blowing the situation out of proportion. She has explained to those close to her that she tends to do this, and they don't need to worry. In a way, by taking responsibility for her behavior, she is empowering herself. By allowing the fantasies to roll, much like a movie unfolding, she is mobilizing her power, power that can be used as self-protection against losses that would overwhelm her—and that did at age four. This is the kind of protection that is common for sensitive people.

Surveying Debbie's childhood clearly sets forth the origins of some of her dramatic creations. When I asked her how she spent her time as a kid, she said, "Imagining." She went on to explain. "I had a pretty restrictive life. We couldn't do much to bother my brother for fear of causing seizures. I had to stay in my room a lot. I would read and imagine myself in the situations I'd read about and take things one step farther. I watched television sometimes, and my bike became My Friend Flicka. Most of my life was pretend."

Debbie smiled the smile of pleasant memories as she described the times she spent imagining. I asked where she lived during her childhood. "It was a very German town with a pretty controlling atmosphere. The community sets standards and if you deviate from them or if your family, parents, or grandparents deviated from those high standards in any way, you were marked. It was like getting put into a little box."

Even more emphatically, Debbie said, "It was a very, very cliquish place to grow up. There was not a lot of information in the sixties about mental handicaps, so there wasn't a lot of understanding about our situation. I don't think people wanted to judge us, but part of their heritage and thinking was that somebody must have done something wrong to cause the situation."

As a response to the constraints and stress of Debbie's early years, she behaved admirably—so much so that she really didn't let her natural personality show a lot. As she mentioned, one of her main coping devices for the distractibility of ADD was to overfocus on whatever she was doing.

Therefore, it comes as no surprise that following a summer job in a county program for children with learning disabilities, she was quickly drawn to the field of special education. Working with the sensory motor development of children in the program felt familiar to her.

Debbie knew something about the neurological basis for what she was studying in high school and "thought it was kind of progressive and pretty neat. From then on," she said smiling, "that was what seemed to come naturally." She had no trouble getting jobs at the state school, and her work and school progressed uninterrupted through two years of college.

Only after moving to Austin for her third year of college did she consider majoring in something else. A bit wistfully Debbie said, "I think I wanted to go into art, but the labs would have taken so much more time and so much more money, and I just couldn't afford it. I had to be practical at that point." She continued working full-time and going to school at the same time. That meant taking the easiest, fastest route possible to a degree.

She noted, "School only became hard when I didn't already know something." Early on her parents exposed her to reading and math, not in a formal way but incidentally at home. High school presented the first time she actually had to study. And that meant trouble when her ADD kicked in. "I couldn't pay attention long enough to really study," she said. "Doing homework was awful. Even though I liked to read, I didn't like to read factual books like history. If the books read more like literature, they would have held my attention.

"Much of my special education learning was hands-on learning. I would experiment on my job using what I was learning in class. That worked great for me. I got to try out everything I was being taught." What Debbie is describing is characteristic of people who have ADD attributes, one of which is a strong tendency to be a kinesthetic learner.

Within the fifteen years after finishing college, Debbie has worked as a special education and early childhood teacher, a special education supervisor, and in an exciting substance abuse-prevention program at Southwest Texas State University.

Throughout her career she's been able to use her creative skills and continues to be excited about the many advantages of working with special kids when you like to *do* things firsthand.

When I First Met Debbie

When a longtime friend invited me to visit the substance abuse-prevention program at Southwest Texas State University, she said, "There's someone you have to meet." That person was Debbie Sager. Little did she know how much we had in common or how long-standing the relationship would turn out to be—or that Debbie would end up in a book I was writing.

We instantly felt comfortable with each other. Now I know it had to do with the magnetic attraction that many people who are ADD feel for each other. (I recall years ago, before I realized how many ADD attributes I have, saying, "I attract people who are ADD like bees are attracted to honey.")

Debbie's background in sensory motor integration, multiple intelligence, and personality theories, and special and early childhood education gave us a common intellectual connection immediately. To this day, we may meet to trade plants for our gardens or for some other reason and end up talking about the relationship between people wired in the ADD way and different forms of intelligence.

How Debbie Envisions the Future

After the Southwest Texas funding dried up, she returned to the public school classroom as an early childhood special education teacher. That was two years ago. She still wonders whether she will ever get back to the type of position she held as a supervisor, where she was responsible for the direction of many children.

Health problems have intervened for her since Southwest Texas lost its funding 1996. She says, "On days when I have good energy, which is more and more of the time now, I think I can get back to the position I was in without the amount of energy I used to pour into my job. I've learned to go with the flow."

Debbie goes on to say, "I believe I'll approach my work as someone who has become deeper and richer with more understanding as a result of having backed up and gotten broader."

But knowing she is ADD has added an additional twist to her plans. "I realize I'm going to have to create an environment, a milieu that fits me," says Debbie. "There are two things I'm discovering. I can work on feeling good about myself on the inside. But I'm learning that I have to create an outside environment that allows me to be comfortable with myself."

Debbie next became specific as she described the environment that she envisions for her future. "I know that a lot of situations like in banks and libraries have a different feel that doesn't support the person I am. For example, though I love books, I hate to go to the library. Any place that is run in a linear, highly organized manner by people who are made the same way doesn't feel very good to me. I don't like to be around them for long periods."

"What I feel good around are action-oriented people, humanistic people who are more interested in helping or having a conversation than in being highly efficient or making the best deal. Shopping is not nearly so much fun as it used to be. And a lot of small businesses that have been personally run are being plowed under by big chains. Even in the small town where I live, efficiency and hair-trigger profits have replaced the kind of personal relationship-based shopping I like. It's hard to find places to shop where I can enjoy a social exchange."

Debbie and her family have recently moved farther out into the country. With twenty-two acres to explore and endless creative ways to use the property to make her dreams happen, Debbie's future has taken on new dimensions. Her gauge for decision-making will depend on how she feels about where she is and what she's doing. "If I feel good somewhere, I'll go there. If I don't, I won't." she says. "I have a reactive personality, and I'm going to use it to create the environment I want."

A dream of Debbie's has been to have a school based on the creative arts. Trying to get it started a year ago didn't work out for her, so she set her dream aside. Now, discovering how important an environment is to her, she has come to the conclusion that it was a very good thing that finding the property and support for the school was delayed.

"My dream is changing a little," says Debbie. "Now I realize that I want to encourage kids to figure out what they need in order to learn to their optimum. It's all part of that self-discipline thing that everybody is touting. But this time it uses the natural strengths that the child has and goes from there. It's training that fits the person."

She continues, "I want young people to know that to be powerful, directed, focused, and self-controlled, you can't learn the way others say you should learn. You can't apply the standards of the society and people who are not wired like you are or who don't think or feel the way you do. You must use tools that fit you to learn and achieve."

"I've had to learn that I don't have to act on the first feelings I have. I had to learn to engage my brain to try to figure out why I'm feeling the way I am and what is making my emotions act the way they are acting.

"*Don't feel ashamed of your emotions. Don't hide them because it's harder to get them back out.*

"I want young people to know that to be powerful, directed, focused, and self-controlled, you can't learn the way others say you *should* learn. You can't apply the standards of the society and people who are not wired like you are or who don't think or feel the way you do. You must use tools that fit you to learn and achieve."

Debbie, the teacher and educational supervisor, has become clear about how she looks at education. Becoming serious, she lowered her eyes and said, almost introspectively, "That's why you can't lay curriculum out six months ahead. You've got to go with the person each step of the way—be individualized.

"You have to educate people so the material fits. And you don't try to work with huge numbers of people. Once you help a child discover how she learns, she can continue to learn using the teacher as needed. To be sure, this is labor intensive in the beginning, but in the long run the children will learn well and thoroughly. Children will learn to ask questions, asking for directions and information instead of having someone coming from the outside attempting to fill their brains with facts and information that have no place in their scheme—creating learning disorder. That's what I want others to know who are younger."

She continued: "I would teach children how to listen to their inner feelings and then to carve their paths. They're in control. They're not going to come off the wall. They will be educated, but in ways that respect how they are made, no matter how that is, and that will allow them to use their talents optimally in the community. Now I'm closer to being ready to create a learning environment that will really be useful to people."

What Works For and Against Debbie

A strongly energetic, bubbly, Outwardly Directed ADD woman, Debbie also has the sensitivity associated with Inwardly Directed ADD. Because she views her ADD as an asset in many situations and has found environments that support the way she is made, Debbie has a long list of positive ADD attributes.

Without hesitation, Debbie tells me, "First off, there's what I used to consider a problem—getting off track if I take a break from what I'm doing. I am learning, though, to allow myself to take a creative break. Then it became an asset. I may work with my plants or concrete [Debbie makes birdbaths and other garden items out of concrete] and still *think* about my job or what I'm going to do the next day."

Debbie considers this a transition phase she's going through. She says, "I can feel it—and it feels great to be able to do something *different* without constantly having to rein myself in.

"Then there's my creativity. I think I am creative," Debbie said with a smile spreading across her face. I nodded affirmatively, also grinning broadly.

Then the smile in her eyes turned dim as she introspectively noted, "You know, it took a long time to allow myself to be creative. I felt I had to fit in to feel safe and accepted. And sometimes, creative people are looked at as eccentric, so I had to link my creativity to the more linear, a more logical methodology. It was always there, but I never gave myself permission to be creative.

"In my town," she explained, "the business people were the ones that were well respected. The work ethic reigned—put your nose to the grindstone. You're seen as flighty and not really dependable and kind of wishy-washy—there one minute and not the next—if you are creative. People gave the impression that you'd never know what would come out of the brain of a creative person. And, finally, it was believed that you couldn't really communicate with creative people because they thought differently."

Debbie analyzed her remarks, "I used to feel very bad about the way I was, but at the same time I couldn't help being the way I was, so I simply hid it. I learned a lot of rhetoric that I could cover my creativity with and became intellectually creative.

"Now I realize that, although I do think differently from many of the people in my hometown—that's my ADD at work—I am also a responsible person who can be trusted. I don't behave in ways that they expect creative people to behave. Best of all, since the time when I worked on my master's degree, I've been able to link things together that don't ordinarily go together. It's been a long time in coming!" Debbie sighed.

There was no hesitation when she talked about sensitivity. "I feel I'm highly sensitive and attuned to other people. That helps me on my job to see what's affecting kids and whether it's affecting them positively or negatively." Debbie doesn't need to test kids or observe them for long periods to know what's going on with them. Her sensitivity is an excellent diagnostic tool that she can use quickly to assess a child's status. It's one she can trust.

Then, having figured out what a child needs, Debbie quickly turns to problem-solving in order to help the child. This, too, is enhanced by her sensitivity because she can think of something, try it out, and ascertain immediately whether it's working. She explained it this way. "When a child doesn't want to try an activity, I can usually figure out why pretty quickly by the feel of his reaction, and I work to make the activity easier." Debbie adjusts her reaction to the child, and the result is a win-win situation for the child, for her, and for others in the environment.

"But sensitivity is not always great, Debbie says. "It can also cause me a world of trouble. I wear my feelings on my sleeve a lot. Recently, I asked my husband for something that rhymed or sounded like 'Loch Ness' (as in the lake creature). He said, 'This house is a mess.' Then, of course, I overreacted. He probably was joking."

Well trained and conscientious, Debbie has discovered methods to work with both of these traits, but it does take effort on her part to stay in control. I want to share how she thinks about these, as she demonstrates a self-forgiving *and* responsible reaction to the downside of her ADD.

In a very matter-of-fact tone, Debbie said, "I'll start with my checkbook. I have trouble with organization in terms of the traditional world that society understands." You'll notice that right away she identifies the problem as one *in relation to the traditional world*. What that means is that she does not feel *bad* or particularly pressured to be able to acquire the skills needed to do that kind of organization well.

She goes on to describe a method for keeping track of her money that she invented many years ago—long before she became aware of her ADD tendencies. It has worked well for her most of the time, so she doesn't normally have any more trouble than someone without ADD attributes.

"Basically I start with a zero balance every pay day. Next I add my deposits. Then I write checks on the back of the checkbook and subtract as I go, rounding off everything to the highest number. At the end of the month, if there is anything left over, I forget about it and actually accrue a little bit of extra money— usually."

Because she can manage her current method, Debbie willingly keeps up with her checkbook. But, she adds, "If I had to do a lot of figuring or was going to try to balance my checkbook monthly, I would just not do it. It's too hard. So, I'll stick with what I will do."

Punctuality is the other area in which Debbie has worked out a creative system of management. Laughing, she quips, "Well, as I walk out the door, there are a hundred million things along the way that need to be done. If I don't allow an extra forty minutes, I'll be late. So I just tell myself that I have to be somewhere forty minutes before I have to be there. That way, I'm on time."

As with all of Debbie's coping skills, she uses her tendency to get sidetracked for a positive outcome. She describes it this way. "As I am ready to leave, I find things on the way to the car that need to be done. I also find that when I get my anxiety level up or my adrenaline up, I can do things more efficiently. As I'm walking out the door, I stop and do this and that, figuring it will only take a second and that job will be done. When I finish that one, I see another which will only take a second. I work very efficiently under these conditions."

I find Debbie's perception of her time management to be

creatively strategic. She has an agenda—all the other jobs she wants to get done. She realizes that under the specific pressure of having to be somewhere on time, she works efficiently. And she has planned how to accomplish both tasks at the same time by simply telling herself she has to leave early. What a wonderful, creative solution to two problems.

Ironically, Debbie has found that after she has practiced her creative solution several times, it becomes rote for her. She no longer has to think about it. So a few days into the school year, she is habituated to planning on leaving her home at 7 A.M. to drive the twenty miles to school, a twenty-minute drive, so that she can arrive at school *on time* for her first class at eight.

Again her strategy works for her, accommodating her ADD so that the areas that could be troublesome really aren't. Debbie is good at taking advantage of an *organizational moment*. Just as the *teachable moment* takes advantage of unplanned circumstances that provide the opportunity to teach, the organizational moment takes advantage of unplanned opportunities to organize or finish a task.

She explains, "It's not methodical, but it works for me. My husband who's not ADD wants me to pick up around the house, one room at a time. Well, if I pick up something in the living room and it goes in the bedroom, and I'm in the bedroom and find something that needs to be done, I go ahead and do it. I accomplish the same thing he does, but not in a methodical way."

As Debbie spoke, I realized that she works exactly the way I do. I think of it as a dance, moving around the house doing a little bit of a lot of things until they all get done. I've noticed that I enjoy this dance and am just as efficient—actually more so than if I were bored to death doing one task all the way through before starting another.

Using a methodical approach, a person does task A for ten

minutes, task B for ten, and task C for ten minutes. Debbie and I do tasks A, B, and C for thirty minutes. At the end we are done and we've had a wonderful dance. It's going with the flow.

Debbie simply reframes what are often considered ADD problems into non-problems by coming up with creative solutions. She lives a way that fits. And it works well for her.

WHAT DEBBIE WANTS YOU TO KNOW

Laugh.

Listen to your feelings.

Learn to differentiate between your first reactive feelings and what you feel at a deeper level.

Remember, no one knows what is best for you like you do—no one else walks in your shoes.

Find out what makes your light burn.

Find your fit, your passion.

Melissa Petty

I like the complexity of ADD. MP

And she enjoys figuring it out to make a wonderful life. LW

The first words out of Melissa's mouth are, "I like the complexity of ADD. To me it always seemed like a jigsaw puzzle that you had in a box that looks strange and doesn't really come together. When you pull all the pieces out, it has meaning for me as an ADD person. It's glorious and grand."

To me, Melissa is a bit of a jigsaw puzzle herself. She appears very feminine, with a soft voice that makes me think of honey and lemon layered with meringue. But watch out! Don't be fooled. She has whimsy sprinkled on top. Then there is the part of her that says, "It's glorious and grand." Her comment comes out emphatically, adding a regal and passionate aspect to her expression. Finally, she's clear minded, intelligent, and able to set good solid limits around herself and what she does.

"In everyday life," she says, "I think of ways in which I used to look disorganized to some degree, and now I realize my life has an organization that fits for me. It just doesn't look as organized as it might for a person who has a certain idea of how organization looks."

You can't pull the wool over Melissa's eyes. She's very clear about what is hers and what isn't. She doesn't buy into the cultural standard for how one should organize a day or live a life. "Sometimes I get up in the morning, and I have no idea what I'll do that day. I don't have the day planned out. I don't put it on a list."

In her matter-of-fact, sweet, yet emphatic tone, Melissa continues, "I have in mind the two or three things that are important to me, and I go from there to put the day together. It's really wonderful to let my ADD free my creativity. And at the end of the day I do get done what I need to do. And it feels right to me, and I feel wonderful.

"Even though I'm an ADD coach, and list making is often subscribed to as very important to ADD people so that they are efficient, I don't keep a lot of lists. I don't subscribe to keeping lists. It doesn't work for me."

Melissa has definitely sorted out what does and does not fit her. She doesn't get caught up in one standard for all. As she says, "I make my life fit for me. One important thing I do for myself is to be self-employed. That works out beautifully.

"I work out of my home where I feel very comfortable. It took years of moving from house to house to house until I found a house with the comfort I want. That means having some green. I can't live in a plot where there's just a house and I see my neighbor through the window. I have to have some green and be able to look out and see some water." I know that Melissa lives in a city in the middle of North Texas, so I wonder where she finds her water. "I have a pool," she explains. "It's concrete water, but it's water. And I have a fountain, because I need to hear the water."

Then, characteristically rephrasing what she'd said. as if to check it out in her own mind, she adds, "So I have some green, and I need some nature and I need some water."

It doesn't take a lot of money or complicated systems to create the ambiance Melissa has obtained. She tells me, "At times when I didn't have a pool, I had a fountain, a small fountain.

One time I just had an old oak bowl filled with water and put some leaves in it."

I wonder how she managed to avoid settling for a house that was less than what she wanted. She explains. "It took a year the last time I bought a house." As usual, she didn't go by a checklist. "I simply looked and searched and the minute I walked in, I knew it was my house. So I just went by the feeling of what fit for me."

Melissa so honors the uniqueness of her way of being that she can count on her inner guidance system to lead her to comfortable outcomes that suit her. She has learned the secret of how to create a designer life that is right for her. And she continually validates the rightness by how her actions feel to her. It hasn't always been that way, however.

Melissa's Background

When I ask about her background, Melissa immediately begins talking about her father. "My father, who carries the genetic ADD line in my family, is a pilot. He was in the military, a typical job for someone like him who is ADD. And one of the things, as I look back, is how beautifully he fit his ADD into his life. And he has had a really happy, successful life. He didn't realize what he was doing, but he was really good at intuitively picking what was good for his life."

Her dad was able to grow up in the country where, as she put it, "He could be gloriously ADD." In contrast, she was raised in the military milieu, going from place to place. Though her mother had a skill of making even the most remote assignment special, Melissa didn't have the freedom afforded her dad.

Similarly, where he had "tons" of family and community around, people who accepted him and thought he was wonderful, Melissa grew up with the Korean War going on and parents who were gone much of the time. Her mother, as the wife of a commander who was head of his squadron, was expected to take care of the wives of other servicemen. Keeping their morale up meant spending a lot of time out her own home.

Melissa's brothers were four and six years younger than she. "I didn't have a lot of choice. The children in the military are expected to be silent and manage their own problems while the father is gone and the mother is taking over." With a bit of humorous sarcasm, she adds, "After all, you can't expect your father who is off saving the world to attend to home."

Melissa bought into the military paradigm. Though she says she "went kicking and screaming," in reality she took over, feeling maternal toward her brothers. To add spice to the situation, they were "pretty active little boys and pretty mischievous. They find it wonderful that I'm ADD, and I find it grand and glorious."

In contrast, Melissa's mother is not considered by the family to be ADD. "She's wonderfully complex, however. She's interesting. She's dramatic. Everything was a drama to her. Even the dullest moments were exciting to her. For example, I didn't realize until much later that an assignment in Minot, North Dakota, was one people hated to receive. My mother made it seem wonderful."

Moving a lot made school tough for Melissa, who was shy, quiet and introspective. Ironically, today, one of Melissa's best skills is in the area of networking and relations with people. But during her early years, she found military kids tough and mean. "And I was not tough and mean," she says. "I didn't know how to take care of myself and deal with teasing."

So many children with ADD wiring, tend to be very, very sensitive. On top of that, we don't initially see the fine points of playground politics. It takes time to figure out the roles that people are playing and then decide what we want to do in relation to them. Arriving at school with open hearts and innocence can quickly turn a sensitive child into a frightened one. That happened to Melissa.

She continues, "Typically, I didn't transition well. Yet there I was changing schools every two years. That was really tough, and it was probably my biggest battle. In response I developed school and social phobias, though I never stopped going to school." She toughed it out, eventually overcoming both phobias completely on her own. She confided, "That's why I went to graduate school in social work—to cure myself."

At that, the twinkle reappears in Melissa's eye and her eyebrows go up as she communicates the delightful self-awareness and insight. "In retrospect, it all makes sense. Not only did I learn that I'm not socially phobic, but I'm just the opposite, very social."

A thought crosses my mind that I share with Melissa.

"Sounds to me like you were an abuse victim." Half expecting that I may have jumped to a conclusion that isn't my business to share, I am relieved at her response.

"I was," she says with a tone to her voice, as if hearing the thought for the first time.

Quickly I add, "The phobic behavior was a protection, not an uncommon reaction for a sensitive ADD kid."

Melissa immediately picks up on my thought, adding, "It was a pretty brutal environment for a sensitive kid. It was brutal for most kids, and it was chaotic, disjointed, and difficult and tougher for me than for many others."

I can't tell you how much I've seen this scenario played out. I'm not talking about abusive parents or intentional abuse. But simply the thoughtless, hurtful teasing and chaos that surrounds many situations where groups of people congregate, like in schools. Add to that the typical military system, not geared to accommodating individual human needs, and you get unrecognized abuse. It's much more prevalent than most people realize. It's just not discussed.

Over time, Melissa feels she did well in school because she developed what she calls an "obsessive-compulsive" side. It helped her get through. Because there is none of it in her family lineage, she thinks she developed the tendencies rather than being born with that chemistry. Then she adds, "The past few years, as I've let go of my obsessive-compulsive behaviors, I have become quite disorganized. I think that's my natural way—to not be obsessive-compulsive."

Then with a smile, she adds, "That doesn't particularly bother me—to be disorganized. In fact, I love it—it's fluid and wonderful. When I was able to let go of the obsessive-compulsive piece, my ADD characteristics came out full blown."

Melissa asserts, "I don't mean that in any negative sense. I would lose things, I couldn't keep up with things, but in no way did I feel that was an imposition on me. I have been enormously freed." By the time she finishes telling me about her release from compensatory obsessive-compulsive behaviors, she's glowing. A look of real happiness radiates from her face, and there is no question but that she means what she says, as she feels her joy clear through to the center of her being.

On the other hand, she doesn't feel sorry she developed the obsessive-compulsive part, either. "It helped me get through school. Probably it would have not been so easy for me to get through college and graduate school if I had not been that way." And, in fact, Melissa worries about the implications of this for her future dream of getting a doctorate. I'm sure she'll solve it, but right now, it is a concern.

With college behind her, she married a lawyer she met when she was thinking about going to law school—although she chose graduate school in social work instead. "I was married and had no idea what to do with myself. Socially phobic, I found the thought of a job terrified me. So I decided to do what I did best. I went to graduate school determined to get a master's degree in social work and overcome some of the things in my life that were a problem. I accomplished both."

She received no help from her family because that's how her family handled finances with the children. "I worked in a beer factory to put myself through graduate school," she says.

More laughter preceded her description of the job. "It was mundane, but I made it interesting thanks to the gift from my mom. I made good money inspecting beer bottles. It gave me plenty of time to think, because I was partially hypnotized by the bottles moving by on the assembly-line belt."

Advanced schooling wasn't very pleasant for this sensitive woman, however. "Graduate school was the most victimizing place in which I ever found myself. The people were the unhealthiest, most dysfunctional, meanest people I ever met.

"There were a couple of professors who verbally abused the students, would use their power to abuse students and would ridicule them if they did something wrong in class. It wasn't even subtle. In addition, they perpetrated a lot of other behavior such as rape, abuse of a student's child, that kind of serious dysfunction."

After graduate school Melissa got a job in a mental health clinic right at the time the state was closing down all the inpatient mental health hospitals in Texas. The patients were dismissed and often ended up on the streets in their home communities. "So, I was right at the beginning of dealing with homeless people. Many of my clients lived under bridges. It was really challenging, and I loved it. I really identified with those people who had difficult times. I thought I was going to be helping them, and I really learned a lot from them. It was a great place to heal."

Melissa used the money she earned for psychotherapy and kept plugging along toward her goal of mapping a way out of her social phobia. Five years later she moved to another job—this time doing geriatric social work for a year. Again she learned. And sadly, again she ran into institutional abuse.

"I found hospitals pretty abusive places to be for employees and patients alike. I learned I'm not very good at the politics of a job. That was what was most difficult for me. It never was the work itself," she says.

Though Melissa could see the office politics operating, she couldn't understand how to play them. She says, "I was extremely aware that they were going on. But there were two problems. I couldn't understand why people did that in the first place. Why not just do your job, and do it well? Secondly, I couldn't figure out why people would want to put their energy into politics. "Though I'm better now at politics, I'm not good at it, and I'll never be. I don't like it. I still don't understand why people want to do it."

I can completely identify with her with regard to her perspective of politics and have heard it often from people who are wired in the ADD way. To me, playing politics feels dishonest, not *real*, which is simply a different perspective on a generally accepted way of operating.

A year in the hospital job was enough for Melissa, but she didn't know what she wanted to do next. "I was kind of like a teenager although I was twenty-eight years old. I experimented with different behaviors.

"While in this period of real flux, I realized I wanted to be a mother. It hit, all of a sudden. But then, what a shock to discover that physically I couldn't be a mom! I went through five or six years of painful infertility and found out how cruel people can be.

"I was incredibly sensitive throughout this time," she says. "But both professional people and family and friends were insensitive. I heard everything from 'Your anger is blocking you from getting pregnant' to people close to me withdrawing. One therapist I went to see about my grief told me I shouldn't feel unhappy. She explained it wasn't as bad as what she had experienced when she had a child die young. Then she added, 'That was a bigger grief.' She denied me my grief and obviously hadn't worked through her own. That's not therapeutic.

"It is an odd position," Melissa said, sharing what she'd gleaned from her experience. "You're trying desperately to do something that other people are trying desperately not to do. It was tough.

"I finally gave up and grieved that I wasn't going to bear a child, and then went through adoption. That was another interesting experience." Melissa laughs as she continues, "Oh, adoption!"

Because Melissa is incredibly resourceful, within six months she left a hospital with a baby boy who was a day and half old. "I hope I can meet his mother some day," she confides. "I'd like to tell her face to face how grateful I am." From the little she's gleaned about her son's birthmother, Melissa feels that she likes her. And she also feels that she, too, is ADD.

Melissa's son is now ten years old. "It has been the most glorious, interesting ride. He's very active and ADD." Chuckling, she adds, "He's a pistol."

She is able to apply everything she's learned for herself and through her work with ADD support groups on behalf of her son.

Melissa lives a designer life—one for which she's been the artistic director. She fully experiences in the present what she needs to learn for her own growth. She has done this by being a mother, wife, professional coach, master's level social worker, ten-year-board member with the Attention Deficit Disorder Association, Southern Region, Cub Scout leader, Sunday school teacher, and school volunteer. Not bad!

When I First Met Melissa

I've known of Melissa for a decade. Beginning in the mid-1980s, I did ADD evaluations for adults at my counseling center and we

met through our work in ADD. I occasionally saw her at conferences, although usually only from a distance. I never really sat
down to talk to her.

When we finally talked in 1996 we found out how many interests we share. I asked her to join me in training professionals to
work with skill building in groups of people who have ADD
wiring. As a result I was able to spend two and half days with her
and saw the Melissa I've come to know. We've shared our similarities and laughed about our differences one of which is our
internal timing.

If I have an idea this minute, I will have had five hundred
thoughts about it by tomorrow, will have made twenty moves,
and will have committed time and energy to doing something to
make the thought a reality, regardless of other projects on my
agenda. Melissa, on the other hand, will think about it, massage
it, and slowly decide what to do, how to do it, and when to do it.

I vividly remember talking with her after she participated in
the skill-building training. She said she definitely wanted to run
a group. The training was at the end of November, and the way
I'm made, I figured she'd run a group in January. Imagine my surprise when she said she thought maybe April or May would be
good for her. She told me she wanted to get a good feel for how
to do the group.

With my spontaneous, high-risk-taking speed and her
thoughtful, well-planned, kneading of the situation, you might
expect that we would have gotten bogged down at that point.
But we didn't. The reason is that Melissa clearly states what she
needs and wants and takes the time to plan for it in her own way.
I understand and accept that Melissa is being Melissa. I realize
she's taking full responsibility for the way she is. I immediately
respect that and don't take her actions personally. Her decisions
are for her, not in relation to me, and have nothing to do with
any inadequacy on my part.

Over the last few months, I've discovered that perhaps more

than anyone I know, Melissa understands with sensitivity the depth of ADD issues. She truly sees the need for change in the way that ADD is formulated and talked about. She knows what it's like to be extremely sensitive in a culture that reflects a linear, judgmental attitude. I look forward to brainstorming and then developing some next steps with her about what to do with what we mutually see as a problem.

How Melissa Envisions the Future

"I see myself moving to where there is more green and more water. I see myself moving to a community of like-minded others: ADD or creative," Melissa says.

She also sees herself pursuing a doctorate, although that is scary to her since she's lost a lot of the compulsive behavior that got her through school before. And she's not willing to recreate that compulsiveness so that it can work for her in the future. Perhaps an alternative doctoral program with more hands-on learning would work well for her. She has a wealth of experience and is perfectly capable of functioning at a higher educational level. But it would be a shame to squeeze this creative, resourceful woman into a little box. So I hope she will go about seeking that higher degree in a creative manner.

A stalwart advocate of finding and living her passion, Melissa says, "Finding your passion sounds so trite and I'm sorry it does because it is so true. I have had to find mine and live it. I must encourage others to find theirs and live it. It's as necessary as drinking, eating and getting yourself clothed."

And again she reiterates, "You have to find it. You have to follow it. And, if you don't, things will not work out, and you'll struggle until you do.

"You'll find it in your own way or have someone point it out to you. I hope you find it. When you do, refine it. That's the key."

Part of Melissa's finding her passion means she will be involved in group activities. "I want to do groups, and I'll always do groups," she says. "I think they are so powerful and healing for everyone, and there is an energy there. Besides I like the companionship of the group. I like the feeling of community.

"I see honoring that sense of community and am drawn to a 'tribal' feeling. That's what I'm trying to do now. I want us in the support group in Dallas to do that for ourselves and for the next generation coming up. That way they will have role models who are forging the way.

"It reminds me of the feminist movement of the sixties. I learned a lot from that. That's my goal for myself and my son. The road won't be as difficult for them. We will have paved a new way for the children.

"I want to help people find someone who is like-minded, probably the same sex, and has gone through the same struggles and is on the same road. That's how mentoring will work. That's a big piece I didn't have. I had to mentor myself. But that would be the biggest key."

What Works For and Against Melissa

Most of what works for Melissa is seen through her outstanding ability to make relationships. Sensitivity leads the list of Melissa's positive ADD attributes, accompanied by compassion, empathy, creativity with networking, and by humor and courage. She loves to use her skills and aptitudes to run groups and work with groups of people. Both interests reflect her strong interpersonal tendency.

Melissa is a good friend to have. She's safe and judgment-free. People like her and her loyalty and stay loyal in return, as long as they are willing to be truthful and take responsibility for themselves.

But, she says, "I no longer have time or interest in anyone who doesn't get the whole picture. I'm tired of putting up with judgmental people who don't see the wonderful uniqueness of all people. I can't abide social politics or role playing. It doesn't make sense to me, and I'm not interested."

Melissa definitely isn't a "couch potato" and wouldn't want to have to work behind a desk. She is always on the go. Her movements are subtle, more like those of a dancer than an acrobat.

Like many ADD people, she is a kinesthetic learner—she learns by doing, not by talking about or thinking about, something. She's done her growing by diving into whatever she encounters. Not one to jump to conclusions prematurely or hide her head in the sand, Melissa faces her struggles directly and courageously while maintaining a gracious, sweet reserve.

She has an entrepreneurial spirit that shows up in subtle form as she brainstorms new ways to change people's attitudes. As a salesperson I doubt you'd find her selling goods, but you will see her selling an idea or a program. Hard sell won't be her approach. Instead, she'll share information and offer her own experience.

With unexpected good humor, Melissa laughs at the paradoxes of ADD—both to teach lessons and for enjoyment. However, she doesn't use humor in a hurtful or sarcastic way. It's not a cover for angry feelings. Rather the humor so characteristic of a healed healer is her style.

At times her lilting giggle makes her sound like a schoolgirl again, though probably one a whole lot more filled with mirth than she was when she was younger. At other times, her laughter sounds like tinkling bells that bring joy to others. There is nothing raucous about Melissa. There's a lot that is joyful. That's self-growth in operation.

Impulsivity is the main problem with which Melissa feels she struggles. Saying things before she takes the time to decide whether or not she really wants to say them sometimes causes her chagrin.

She also finds she spends a lot of time looking for things. Although she says that doesn't really bother her much, she also says, "If I didn't have to spend so much time looking, I'd be able to get to more of the many things I want to do. There are so many people I want to be with that some of those small things get in my way a little bit."

And she still has some secondary problems related to being wired in a way that is not honored by others. "I still have some problems feeling ashamed if I do attempt something that I feel inadequate doing." She says softly, "My family is very much into looks and what looks good. I still have a little piece of me that, if I look a little bit 'flaky' or I get distracted for a minute or I say something to someone that is unkind and that I didn't mean— being impulsive—I feel bad about it."

Becoming introspective, Melissa continues, "That's the worst part for me, hurting someone inadvertently because I am distracted. Or when I say something that I don't mean to say— before I think. I suffer."

In her inimitable fashion, Melissa is working on coping with these characteristics. "I have a plan to deal with them. I explain to the other person what happened. I don't make excuses, but I explain. I ask forgiveness, and I make amends. And then I go on.

"I realize that I'm not going to cure my speaking out or unwittingly hurting of someone. But I've discovered that everybody else in my life is a whole lot more understanding about that than I am, and they give me a lot of leeway." Yes, ADD people can be tough on themselves! But Melissa is learning to be kind to herself and advises other to follow suit.

Choosing the type of life she wishes to live has put Melissa in charge of her environment. And she purports to keep it that way. She chooses to be around like-minded people, people interested in learning more and growing more and in being themselves. "I'm not worried about being conventional," Melissa says with a big smile on her face. "And I don't see that for my son, either. I have learned to enjoy being an ADD woman."

Feeling grateful is probably the result of her resourcefulness in mastering situations and making something good out of whatever she finds. Her mother's lessons run deep. Because of this, she simply doesn't look at herself as having ADD problems.

WHAT MELISSA WANTS YOU TO KNOW

Go find a mentor.
Be kind to yourself and others.
Find the passion in your life.

Bill and Sharon Larson

I keep getting overwhelmed. There's so much to do. BL

Bill underestimates himself. SL

And together, they get the job done. LW

From the very beginning, I planned to tell Bill and Sharon Larson's story from the angle of their relationship. Bill is ADD, and Sharon, his wife, is not. Together their stories provide a clear picture of ADD relationship issues. Ironically, the very first thing out of the mouth of each was about the other.

"Sharon went to work as an R.N. with the medical practice I worked with in 1977," Bill says. "I was pretty dysfunctional at the time in relation to where my personal life was going—you know, disorganized, impulsive, procrastinating—all the classic ADD problems. Work was easy. The rest of my life was a mess."

Sharon's first words to me are, "I think he kind of underestimates himself. He's probably one of the best known physicians in Anchorage, Alaska—been there thirty years." To this, Bill's response is, "It's a good thing I practiced in Anchorage all that time. If I'd skipped off and been a gypsy like many of my ADD patients are, I would have led a really dysfunctional life. Who knows where I'd be now!"

Insightfully, Sharon observes, "Many doctors who ended up in Alaska in the early days were probably ADD." She is referring to Alaska's special lure for adventurers, many of whom are ADD. "Bill is like them, a very hands-on, caring type person, who has a reputation of being a maverick because he is willing to be himself."

Does this sound like casting for an ADD story?

Bill begins his history talking about his clutter. Over and over, he talks about being overwhelmed by the mess around him—the paper mess. Here's how the story goes from Bill's perspective. "The clutter was the catalyst for the two of us splitting up the first time we tried to live together back in 1979–1980.

"One evening, after having all my newspapers, magazines, and everything I was reading all over the house—including the living room, kitchen, dining area, and bedroom—Sharon announced that the family was thinking of moving. True, I'd left everything in a chaotic fashion, undoubtedly looking like a God-awful mess."

It seems that Sharon was feeling overwhelmed by the mess. As she puts it, "We made the perfect doctor-nurse duo. Bill just dropped whatever he was reading when he was through with it, leaving his mess for 'the nurse' to come along and pick up. But, I was 'off duty' at home and didn't like the job.

"Add to that the fact that my two kids, five and seven, and his teenagers, fifteen, seventeen, and nineteen, made a lot of bodies to fit in with all that paper. However, that's not all. The seventeen-year-old's girlfriend was there all the time. The nineteen-year-old and her girlfriend moved in and out according to finances. The fifteen-year-old son was home holidays and during the summer.

"His daughter and I were fed up. So we concocted a plan. We'd given Bill a parrot for his birthday. He adored the bird. His daughter was going to spend the night at a girlfriend's and I said, 'Take the parrot with you.'

"That night at dinner, Bill noticed the bird was gone and asked where it was. I said, 'The bird has had it. The bird's left home. He can't deal with this mess any more.' Bill looked at me and asked, 'Where's Shura (his daughter) ?'. I said, 'She went with the bird.' He asked, 'Where are your kids?' and I said, 'Well, they're not here.'"

In retrospect Bill realizes that Sharon was "tweaking" him just a bit. But at the time he reacted, big time. His version of the story describes what happened next. "I just blew my stack. My anger management and temper control weren't very good. I went racing around the house picking up stuff like a madman. I was throwing it in trash cans and kind of out of control."

Sharon confirms Bill's reaction. "He came down with his fist on the dining room table and said, 'All right!' Then he stood straight up. Out came the garbage bags. He was like a tornado going through the house."

Retrospectively, Bill is more self-deprecating about how he "used to be" than Sharon is critical. He says, "I was obviously in denial, 'There's nothing wrong with me. I'll fix the problem right now. I'm really upset about this. I haven't done anything wrong except for a few papers strewn around the house.'"

In contrast, Sharon adds humorously, "He picked up everything, that's for sure. There was no trash or garbage to be seen. Granted it only lasted for a week!"

Continuing, Sharon assures me, "It was a side I'd never seen in him before. I'd never seen him very angry. I didn't fear for my own bodily damage, but," she adds, again laughing, "I didn't know if I'd be in the garbage bag."

This description of home life was not much different from her first impression when she walked into his office in 1977. "There were so many unpacked boxes around the office that I asked him if they'd just moved in. I discovered that they'd been there for eight months.

"I was so impressed, though, by this six-foot-one-inch man

sitting on the floor trying to make friends with a two-year-old that I forgot about the boxes, drawn by his warmth and generosity with people. I never forgot the image of the piles all around, but I didn't think about the implications of them when we decided to live together."

That period of their romance lasted only two years from 1978 to 1980. Then they separated, and each married and divorced other people before finding what Bill calls "a wonderful journey—a fairy tale kind of thing." With his voice trailing off, he now says, "I can't imagine being with a more wonderful person."

They started seriously seeing each other again after remaining friends for ten years. Getting romantically back together in 1990, they married, finally, in 1994.

So how did these two people finally manage to make it together in life? Let's look at their backgrounds, their attraction, and the final success of their relationship.

Bill and Sharon's Backgrounds

Both Bill and Sharon were "good little kids." Both were quiet. Both were compliant children. Both had half sisters. Bill's were much older, and Sharon's half sister was younger. But the similarities end there.

Bill's parents stayed together. He describes his father as "older," in his forties and stable, having sown his wild oats and "had his motorcycle accident" before marrying. His mother, whom Bill describes as "very organized and very German," kept track of Bill's many interests. As a member of the Boy Scouts— and reaching three levels beyond Eagle Scout—Bill found a place to express his different interests by earning merit badges with the help of his mother's capacity to keep him on track. She would tell him, "Let's finish this one up," when Bill would flit to a new interest before finishing the last one.

Sharon's parents, in contrast, divorced when she was twelve. Though her mom could be a lot of fun, the pressures of being divorced in a small, southern town at that time made it very hard for her and Sharon. Not owning a car and not having much money, they stayed mostly to themselves. Sharon's reaction? "It was pretty boring."

Her father could be jovial, but you never knew what to expect, and he often would switch emotions quickly. With her own emotion still showing in her voice after all these years, Sharon says, "He was Scrooge. He wasn't physically demonstrative. He took out his anger at mom and the divorce on me. He was never there for me." This colored Sharon's attraction to the opposite sex when she reached adulthood, she says. "I was drawn to men who are demonstrative, who are always doing things and are sensitive, because I like their energy."

Laughingly she says, "All three of my marriages were to ADD men. I've had one husband of each type. My first was bouncing off the wall. An outwardly expressive person, he brought experiences into my life that I never had before. My second husband was also a doer, but he was a nitpicky doer. 'Do things my way, the right way, or do them your way, the wrong way,' he'd say. This approach eventually destroyed us. We hiked, did lots of outdoors activities and active things, but I couldn't live with the critical pressure."

Sharon is very honest about what she has gotten from her ADD spouses. "I found that to be the person I am today, I thrived on being around people who are ADD. I love their energy. I love the thought of being a part of that, because I don't have the capability in myself to generate a lot of these things. Being around folks that are ADD really makes life interesting and exciting. I love it," she says. As I listen to Sharon describe the broadened horizons introduced by her husbands, I watch her glow.

"There's still the same excitement with Bill," she says. "Bill, who's basically laid back, epitomizes the quiet ADD person who is a helper sort. That's important to me. I also like the romanticism of the doctor-nurse duo who help those in need." With maturity, both have learned to value each other, to appreciate each other, and "to own their own emotional stuff." As Sharon says, "It took some trial-and-error learning for us to get this relationship stuff right."

Much of the conversation with Sharon and Bill centers around what was once Bill's practice but has become their joint practice. They have arrived at this point consciously, each having started out going in a different direction and each having stood independently of the other, "paying their respective dues" and gaining experience that they now use jointly.

Originally trained as a registered nurse in a three-year program, Sharon returned to school in 1975 to get her bachelor's degree in nursing with a minor in mental health. But upon graduating, her desire to work in public health bumped up against a hiring freeze in public health, so she ultimately went to work in the clinic where Bill practiced.

Her varied background includes teaching childbirth education and being a substitute school nurse. In the mid-1980s she earned a master's degree in counseling and enjoyed doing crisis intervention. She also spent eight years in gynecology, during which time she volunteered with the rape crisis program. From there she finally made it into public health, working for six years in a clinic that treated people with sexually transmitted diseases. She's also certified in health education.

As a young doctor, Bill thought he might go into internal medicine but realized how much he liked pediatrics during his internship. He tells me, "Internal medicine had too many details, too many long interviews with patients who came in with bags of medication and histories that went back, it seemed, forever. It just overwhelmed me. I enjoyed the free spirit and happier attitude of 'peds' and pediatricians."

Sharon lovingly points out that Bill is also a board-certified pediatrician who also specializes in allergy. He considers that specialty to be a diversion from ADD. It was from Sharon that I learned that Bill is recognized as an authority on ADD, with thirty years' experience working with kids wired in the ADD way.

Like many of us, Bill originally became interested in the subject because of his own child. At three, his youngest child was diagnosed with minimal brain dysfunction (an old term for ADD). "You name it, he did it," was the description given for Bill's hyperactive, impulsive son. Placed on medication, the child has grown into a thirty-three-year-old man who works on the Alaskan pipeline. As Sharon puts it, "A perfect job for him. He's great."

Bill's two older children, both girls, have not been officially diagnosed with ADD but have lots of highly structured ADD traits. So Bill got his first exposure to ADD on a personal level.

By staying in the practice of pediatrics for as long as he has, he has also watched the ADD kids he worked with grow up. And they did not leave their ADD behind, although they were told they would "outgrow it." He continues to see them as teens and through their college years.

Sharon says, "When all the publicity started hitting about adult ADD, we just kind of fell into it—but very cautiously." They worried because controlled substances, such as Dexedrine, are used to treat ADD and their use is carefully monitored by the state and federal government. The fear of drug abuse by patients loomed as a threat initially as adults began to be treated for ADD.

Their worries proved groundless. Sharon comments that out of the thousand or so ADD adults they've seen since the early 1990s, only a very few caused them concern in relation to misuse of medication.

Out of their professional involvement with ADD, Bill began to observe his own behavior. Several times he commented to Sharon, "I think I'm more ADD than this person I just said was ADD." And Sharon agreed with him.

"I was delighted to hear his observation," she says. "Frankly the first couple of years we were back together, I wondered if I'd jumped back in the fire again. But the more he noticed his ADD and began to attend to it, the more he settled down."

Sharon, too, "began to see some of the crazy stuff Bill said and did in the past in a new light." With this understanding, she adds, "More importantly, like I tell some of the non-ADD spouses or 'significant others' I see in the office, I no longer take some of Bill's behavior or lack of it personally, the way I did in the past. That doesn't mean I don't get angry and upset with him. I just don't take it personally."

The icing on the cake was Sharon's comment, "When he asked me to marry him four years ago, I was ready to say yes. If he'd asked me five years ago, I couldn't have done it."

When I First Met Bill and Sharon

Surrounded by eager people all talking at once, I was struck by the calm atmosphere that Bill and Sharon brought onto the stage in Anchorage, Alaska, in 1997. I'd just done an evening presentation about ADD after a couple of grueling days of working within a small group session. I had a headache and was feeling a tremendous amount of stress. It was on this trip that my nerves snapped about the issue of ADD being pathologized and medicalized to death.

Worst of all, I felt as if I were surrounded by a sea of people who thought very differently than I did. My own strength had been sapped trying to get people to understand that ADD is not a "disorder." I'd been trying, somewhat fruitlessly, to explain how it is made a problem in a non-ADD culture where people either fail to receive training in the way in which they learn or are expected to do things in ways that don't fit.

Frustrated and angry, I breathed a sigh of relief when Bill came up and responded warmly with understanding. Then I realized that Sharon, too, got my message and that they were trying to deal with people on a very practical level, helping ADD adults build down-to-earth skills to deal with their ADD in a non-ADD environment. What a relief!

Since that time, Bill and Sharon have become group trainers in my ADD skill-building program. They have immersed themselves in really trying to help their patients learn to utilize the advantages of their ADD while getting the liabilities under control.

Bill says it well. "Medication improves focus, wakefulness, and alertness and reduces distractibility and impulsivity. However, if people don't work on other aspects such as disorganization, time mismanagement, and procrastination, they're not going to go anywhere in life with their ADD. We've decided we're not going to take on patients who aren't willing to do other things to help themselves besides take medication. That's a firm decision!"

How Bill and Sharon Envision the Future

Prior to their marriage, Bill was feeling stressed about his future and burned out. And as a result, his future looked pretty bleak. Now he and Sharon are excited, having made the decision recently that rather than retiring and doing something else, they will spend another ten or fifteen years practicing, which would put Bill into his late seventies.

Neither Bill nor Sharon is a thumb twiddler. In addition, the word *excitement* came up as each spoke of the future. They really love their work with ADD. And they like working together.

Feeling fulfilled in her own right, Sharon is quite ready to settle in with Bill and work with ADD, which will utilize a lot of her counseling and teaching skills. But retire? No way!

What Works For and Against Bill and Sharon

First of all, I've noticed how willing Bill is to "just be human." That is refreshing for someone with as many credentials and as much experience as he has accumulated. He has a naivete about his achievements, especially his personal growth, that catches one off guard.

Like many Alaskans, Bill fits his rugged environment and has thrived, in part, because of his ADD style of brainwiring. He's empathetic in addition to being adventurous and energetic. But it's Bill's ability to work within a structure that got him through medical school. It's also what helped him fit into Boy Scouts. Typically, he's had to rely on the structure of the curriculum or upon acceptable standards and procedures to succeed, just as in childhood he relied on his mother to keep him on task with his scout work.

Logic helps Bill know what to do in medicine, where the practices are specific to the situations. He is very bright and so has done well by choosing a specialty that allows for a lot of variability, joking around with the kids, and opportunity to demonstrate his compassionate nature in a healthy environment. Working with ADD people means working with many of the same characteristics. Dealing more with health than illness, he finds his high sensitivity level is not overstressed. Having a second subspecialty as an allergist keeps Bill from getting bored.

"Being an allergist is kind of a Sherlock Holmes thing—we're always searching for the culprit!" he says.

He admits, however, to having very much enjoyed his 1970s experience as an emergency room physician at night and on weekends. As he says, "It was the classic high stress job! You get to do twenty things at once and that kept me from getting bored. It both used my ADD ability to react quickly and soothed my ADD tendency to get bored." Bill is good at what he does because of his ADD, not in spite of it.

In his marriage, because of his sensitivity and caring nature, he has been able to put in the work he needs to develop habits that he missed developing early on. Though his marriage history isn't necessarily pretty, he's received his lessons on the job, so to speak—hands-on learning. And now at age sixty-one, he's growing. How wonderful not to be stuck in habits that are self- or other-destructive. It's his ADD sensitivity that has made it possible for him to respond to a woman in a way that creates a "wonderful marriage." Good for you, Bill!

Sharon feels, "We have one of the best marriages there ever was. We have put forth the energy to keep it as perfect as we can. We must not let things build. In the past Bill would keep things in and then would blow. Now, because of not being sure how we might have heard one another, we stop."

Sharon's example will sound familiar to many ADD spouses. "This just happened. I was to clog [dance] at a fair out of town where we were headed for some R & R. I came in the evening before we were to leave and announced at dinner that my group was going to get together earlier the day of the fair to practice."

"Bill became upset, saying, 'You've never practiced just prior to a show. Why this time?' It seems he was planning to take me clamming two hours before the show! He was quite tired, acting like the hurt 'little boy.' I left him sitting in his office where he proceeded to pout!

"I was upset. This show was the primary reason for the trip. We were to leave early the next morning. 'Terrific!' I thought. I knew his feelings were hurt, and so were mine. The simplest way was not with words—they would never work at this point. Instead of talking, I put on a sexy nightie. The next morning, all was resolved." At that point Sharon gives a big smile. (And Sharon got her clogging practice in and they went clam digging later.)

But Sharon has also had to learn to talk openly. "We've talked about the basic differences between men and women and then added the ADD stuff to that. I know when I have to be more tuned in to Bill's cues, picking up on whether he's really hearing me. For example, if he's tired at the end of the day or has a lot on his mind. It's times like that it's easy to get into a wrangle.

"I know that if I tell him something and he doesn't respond, I have to watch what I say. I could easily say, 'I told you that,' and he'd say, 'No, you didn't.' I'd say, 'Yes, I did,' and we'd be off to sure defeat.

"I've learned to be more aware of when his wheels are going so he may not be listening to me. Picking the appropriate times when I know I have his undivided attention has been an important lesson for me to learn. I know when we can talk about things that are very important to me."

She continues, insightfully. "It's not a matter of my things not being important to him. That's what I used to think. I understand that it's also not so much that I'm not important to him, but that he's on another tangent that's sparked him to think about something else, and he's gone. I didn't realize this with my first and second husbands."

Bill and Sharon give identical answers to the question about what causes trouble for them. Both say, "We're working too hard."

Though this in and of itself is not an ADD problem, it used to become a problem because of ADD. Bill now handles the work pressure differently. He tells how he recently handled such stress.

"I said "Sharon, we have to talk, because our practice has gone nuts.' In the past I'd have begun to obsess about it, which is a gut-wrenching feeling. Then I would have exploded with my neck muscles becoming rigid and my gut turning over. If I hadn't been able to talk to Sharon about this, it would have eventually gone away, but I would have had a horrible, horrible time.

"Instead of letting it build and build, hitting me one evening when I felt the world collapsing all around me, I stopped. This time I felt let down because I'd overcommitted myself, but I still stopped. And I said to Sharon, 'Let's talk!'"

Listening to Bill, I wonder how Sharon viewed the patient overload. It turns out that she, too, was bothered by it. Neither Bill nor Sharon likes to keep people waiting for two and three months to be evaluated. They both care enormously for the people seeking help.

Interestingly, she also did not see the overload coming. Unlike Bill, however, she didn't beat up on herself. She thought about the situation strategically, wondering how to get other physicians involved and how to plan ways to speed up service while maintaining high quality.

When I ask them for another example of a problem related to ADD, Sharon responds, "Let me give you an example that's happening right now—one in which I'm ready to kill. My mother arrives in a little over two weeks. Her room is Bill's home office. You stand at the door and get a glance at the bed." At that she laughs heartily and continues, "It's probably going to be a few minutes before my mother arrives that he'll get in there going after things."

Sharon confides that there are times when she bites her lip to keep from saying, "I told you so. If you'd gotten with the program, this wouldn't be happening." But she's learning and he's getting it, too, when he "gets behind the eight ball" and feels frustrated.

Together, Bill and Sharon are understanding and conquering the impact of ADD in their lives. And by the work they're doing, they're learning how to help others.

WHAT BILL AND SHARON WANT YOU TO KNOW

FROM BILL

Learn about ADD.

Read about ADD.

Think positively about ADD.

Get an evaluation.

Be sure to see someone who really knows a lot about ADD.

Look for the positive.

Work on the negatives

Accept the reality of the person you are.

FROM SHARON

Read practical books on communication.

Attend a support group together.

Get counseling as a couple—be sure to choose a counselor knowledgeable about ADD.

Accept and understand ADD issues.

Do not take this whole thing so personally.

Realize that your spouse may not be able to be "fixed."

Look for the positives.

Work on the negatives.

Kelly Burkey and Deb Ohnesorge

I think in round-about ways compared to other people. KB

Kelly is floored at the amazement his co-workers have over
his ability to solve practical problems. DO

And his round-about ways lead to creative problem-solving
par excellence. LW

Wiggling toes and twitching fingers characterize Kelly Burkey, a
thirty-three-year-old childlike ADD man whose daughter at age
two shows definite signs of having inherited her dad's ADHD
(attention deficit hyperactivity disorder)—the hyperactive vari-
ation of attention deficit disorder.

One thing's for sure: when you come anywhere near Kelly, you
know instantly that he is very, very physically active. But he's
not offensive. During our interview, he tells me, "Sitting still is
hard for me so I wiggle my toes back and forth in my shoes. My
fingers move all around. My hands do all kinds of awkward
motions. Most times I can't keep myself still. After sitting a little
while, I start moving everything."

I remember a little over a year ago when Kelly was taking an
anger management class, he had to sit still for two hours twice a
week. When I asked how he managed, he instantly pulled a toy
out of his pocket to show me. Showing me rather than answering
my question with words, he produced a liquid bubble toy in a

tube that makes no noise when it's twisted and turned. That's a good thing since even while showing it to me, he constantly manipulated the toy.

It worked in the class and it works any other time he needs to discharge the kinetic energy that quickly builds up inside him when he's sitting.

I know Kelly quite well, and he knows I don't care if he sits, stands, or moves around the room when we are together. He did all three while we talked. The throw rug by the couch where we sat was a bit wrinkled when he left. He demonstrated his active "toe-pointing" mannerism that always gives him, his "committed other" Deb Ohnesorge, and me a good laugh.

Deb and Kelly tease, but in a nonhostile, joyful way. Not long into the interview, Deb pops up and says, "You know, Kelly's hyperactivity has really rubbed off on me. Now I find that I point my toe just like he does when I'm restless or trying to underscore something important."

At that, she sticks her right foot out and to the back with a little weight resting on the pad. "He does this when he's restless and talking and playing. It's just Kelly. Now, it's me, too."

With Deb's support, Kelly has gotten started on a career track—one that means he's stayed on a job longer than ever before, one that he likes, and one in which he has a good chance of succeeding.

Employed by a small-town public works department, he spends most of his time outside. His job provides him with a great big playground. He trims trees, runs heavy equipment, and is currently building a riverwalk. Every day is different for Kelly. His co-workers are amazed at his ability to eyeball a job and, without instruments, accurately construct a walkway with angles all in the right places.

Just the other day, he says, "My boss and another guy were laying out a part of the walk. Precise measurements of distances were required so they had to keep track of the numbers involved.

They hollered a figure out and then forgot about it, whereas me, I grabbed that figure and stuck it in my brain, you know, stick it where I'm standing, and continued to work. About twenty minutes later, they say, 'What was that number we were supposed to remember?' I just yell the figure out. Everyone on the crew looks at me like I'm crazy. They check it, and sure enough, yell back, 'He's right.'"

Kelly's ADD is an asset at work. He says, "I do pretty good because we have seven projects going on at the same time. I can keep all of it together in my mind when everybody else is going crazy running around like a chicken with its head cut off." At that, Kelly laughs loudly, partly proud of what he can do—a pride that has been long in coming—and partly insightful about how useful a trait that previously seemed negative can be.

When I ask Deb for a representative sample of Kelly's ADD, she chortles and says, "When we drive together and his hand is constantly moving all over mine, I know all about his ADD. We don't just hold hands. He's constantly rubbing over me. He goes up my arm, back to my finger, and around my wrist. Fortunately I like it."

Kelly dropped out of high school in the tenth grade and hasn't been back to school since. Many of the intervening years have been tough for him until he discovered his ADD at age thirty-one and, almost simultaneously, developed a relationship with Deb. Since then, he's make enormous strides toward stabilizing his life and finding the opportunities to use his talents and innate intelligence to his advantage.

Kelly and Deb's Backgrounds

Born and raised in Montana, Kelly has two sets of half brothers, ranging in age from eighteen to thirty-three. However, he was raised pretty much as an only child until he was nine, spending most of his time with his mother's parents. Of this arrangement, he says, "I enjoyed the heck out of it. I was irrigating the field when I was seven. I drove tractors and generally was free to do everything even though it drove my grandfather crazy."

What did this rambunctious "troublemaker" do that he now laughs about? Consider the day he made a landing pad in a stack of hay. Kelly tells it this way. "I figured it would be fun to jump out of Grandpa's truck on the way home. Beforehand, I'd picked a good spot and fixed up some bales of hay at the side of the road so I'd have a good landing pad to jump onto. The pad was five or six feet wide, and I knew I wouldn't get hurt when I fell into it.

"I was riding in the back of the truck with my grandpa at the wheel. Grandpa was cruising along the farm-to-market road, traffic going back and forth, doing maybe forty or fifty miles per hour, when all of a sudden he said he 'seen legs.' I flew out the back of the truck."

Deb chimes in at this point with amazement in her voice. "Why did you do that? It was obviously premeditated. Why did you do that? I'd have had to kill you."

Without hesitation, Kelly, with a big grin on his face says, "I was always doing shit like that." In reality, Kelly looks pretty proud of the trick he played on his grandpa. And he looks mighty happy with the response he got from Deb.

With both Deb and Kelly laughing, she continues, "First he'd have to see that you were all right and then he'd have had to kill you."

"Not really," says Kelly. "He said he didn't realize I was gone. He just saw legs. He saw something out of the corner of his eye. And he thought it was something blowing out of the truck and never bothered to stop. He got around the corner, 'bout a quarter of a mile to the house and grandma said, 'Where's Kelly? Where's Kelly?'

"I was lying in the hay, happy. I didn't care. I was playing with the mice and the cats. I was probably nine." Kelly didn't really think that qualified him as a troublemaker. "No," he says, "That was having fun to me. But my grandma didn't see it that way. Grandpa, however, taught me to drive and laugh a lot."

From the warmth and caring he received from his grandparents, Kelly learned to be gentle handling the farm animals— like when he milked the cows. "You just don't pull hard on them, jerking their teats. Grandpa taught me how to milk gently." Kelly proceeds to demonstrate how he'd been taught to use his fingers, not his whole hands, to milk. By the time he finished demonstrating, I thought I might even be able to milk a cow.

Kelly has other family members who are also ADD, with lots of hyperactivity. "My whole family's pretty much ADD," he says. "One of my half brothers is good with mechanics, another is kind of computer-y. Yeah, that's it. He's computer generated." As indicated, his daughter already shows signs of having ADD attributes, and his mom, in all probability, passed the ADD wiring along to her son and granddaughter.

However, Kelly's mom is not eager to embrace the whole idea of ADD. Kelly says, "She told me, 'You're crazy, Kelly. There ain't none of us sick but you.' I tried to explain to her, 'It's like Mom, you don't understand. This ain't something I grew into. This ain't just something, this disease that I grasped.'" At that, he reaches out with his hand, grabbing a bunch of air. Then he continues, "I told her, 'This came in my genes. Your genes.'"

Remembering the conversation with his mother makes Kelly grin just a little. But his grin fades as he recalls his school experiences. "I was secluded and left out," Kelly says. He talks about how he was put off in a corner or left alone because he couldn't sit still. Math, especially, came to Kelly's mind as a problem—not because he couldn't do it but because he couldn't follow the teacher's guidelines.

"You see," he says, "I couldn't keep my attention on the blackboard long enough to wait to write the problems down or be called on. Instead I already had the answer in my head most of the time. She would put formulas on the board and I would look at 'em and have an answer, and I wouldn't write it down.

"As a result, the teacher said I was defiant because I was supposed to write the problem down on a piece of paper and figure out what the answer was. Yeah, I got the label 'Oppositional-Defiant' put on me. I couldn't understand that. I told her, 'You already wrote it down up there. Why do I need to write it down again?'"

Kelly dropped out of school, took his GED right away, and in six months went into the service. When I ask him what the service was like, he answers, "Hell. But not the kind of hell you might think. It was pen, pencil, and pad hell. It had to be this way. Order. I got order in my life, but not their order. Some of the stuff they wanted me to do was stupid."

They gave Kelly rank and then took it back right away. He had trouble getting along with supervisors, trouble with people telling him what to do. "Now," he says, "as I've gotten older, I realize the problem I really had was the way they told me to do things. Their mannerism, their tones. It wasn't what they were asking me to do that caused me the trouble. It was the way in which they told me to do it."

Trained as a hydroelectric and turret mechanic, Kelly was in for a big shock when he tried to transfer his skills to civilian life. That didn't work very well. "I either had too much experience or not enough," he says. "I got where I'd ask, 'How dumb do you need me to be? I need a job.'"

Only once did he end up at a desk job. "That about killed me." he recalls. "I couldn't sit behind a desk. I had been installing and servicing appliances. I was doing good. But I could also talk to people so they put me into sales. I lasted a week. Somewhere between twenty and thirty jobs later, Kelly ended up in the mobile-home business. He sometimes worked for himself and sometimes worked for other small companies.

Only in the last year has Kelly found a job that he really

likes—one in which he seems to be thriving. Previously he really didn't have a career plan. But settling down with Deb, dealing with his ADD, completing a divorce from his daughter's mother, and taking responsibility for his daughter, Kelsie, have changed Kelly. He seems to have shifted into a new chapter in his life—that of a stable citizen. Kelly now has the age and experience behind him to understand a whole lot that he had not picked up earlier. He's found a good job fit and he is able to see hope for his future.

Kelly has begun to write poetry and draw pictures, on the side, primitive in nature, his sensitivity and talent showing through. Polishing his craft will come over time. He looks forward to a time when he can buy art supplies and begin to take some night classes.

Kelly is what I call an undereducated person. Smarter than is suggested by the number of years of education he has managed to accumulate, he likes to read about a wide variety of subjects as well as watch educational programs on television. He soaks up information like a sponge. And he is a willing student now.

Deb has led a very different life. She, too, is finding her way with Kelly's help, to feel good about herself. While she gives information and experience to Kelly, he gives her emotional sup-port that's helping her finally achieve her potential.

The oldest of four children, Deb grew up in Texas, first in Amarillo and then in Lubbock. Right after high school, she spent three years at Texas Tech University majoring in child develop-ment and food and nutrition. She didn't finish college because her husband was transferred to Germany in the armed forces.

Growing up, she was the "mother" to her brother, two years younger. Their dad had died when the children were pre-schoolers and Deb took over. Another brother and sister were born after her mother remarried. Deb continued to take a lot of responsibility for all the children. Tagged by her own mother with the phrase, "Mother of the World"—said in a rather derogatory tone—Deb as a child spent time playing with friends and reading when she wasn't caregiving.

At twenty-three, Deb became a widow and found herself spinning from the turn of events in her life. She moved to Austin, Texas, and stayed single only a year before meeting the man who would become her husband for twenty-two years. Her divorce came after being battered by her husband for several years, in large part in relation to their alcohol usage.

Now forty-eight years old, she's still struggling with a tendency to be the caretaker of the world. But she's doing a whole lot better taking care of herself than she used to. She's learning, though the hard way.

Long ago while in Germany, Deb experimented with drugs. She says, "I never went out on the street to get them." Very socially aware and unwilling to do anything socially inappropriate, Deb has always tended to use drugs and alcohol because "they were readily available."

After the death of her first husband in an automobile accident, she hung with a crowd in Austin that provided her with drugs again. But it wasn't until 1989 at the age of thirty-eight that she got into drugs and alcohol in earnest. "In part I was self-medicating to avoid feeling the pain of being a spousal abuse victim. In part, chemical abuse had become a habit."

But in 1993, at the time she finally left her second husband, Deb stopped cold turkey when two friends came up to her and said, "You can't let this happen to you." Deb says, "I'll never forget that night. I was working, in front of an audience of people I knew. That's when these friends came to me, right there in the middle of everything."

Modestly and quietly, Deb explains, "They were not only responding to my badly bruised face, but to the blackout I'd suffered after the previous night's drinking. I couldn't remember a thing. But I think they must have either seen me or heard about what happened. I don't remember.

"I was scared into sobriety. A DWI didn't get me to stop, but my friends sure could." And Deb's been sober ever since. She still helps people and has a very soft heart for anyone who is trying. But she can look a person in the eye, having "been there, done that," and can "call them on their bullshit!"

When Deb and Kelly met, Deb had begun to build a responsible life for herself. Despite her tough history, she is well respected in the small Central Texas town where she's lived for nearly two decades. Kelly saw the true Deb beneath her history and responded to her immediately. His ADD sensitivity allowed him to see what was really there.

And Deb saw a light in Kelly that many might not have noticed at the time. She knew he had a good heart. She does, after all, read people well. And Kelly hasn't disappointed her. He has learned from her.

Fifteen years Kelly's senior, Deb has taught him a lot of simple, everyday life things that he'd never been exposed to before. He in turn has given her the warmth, affection, unconditional love, and acceptance she has needed but not experienced for so long that she's almost forgotten how it feels.

Kelly loves to take care of Deb and protect her, turning the tables on the one who always did that for others. It's really sweet to see the smiles on their faces as she allows him to help her and he feels the pride in feeling adequate. Perhaps for the first time in their lives, they have a chance to grow whole.

When I First Met Kelly

Every year, the town of Bastrop, Texas, puts on a community program called Yesterfest in late spring. Many of us in the community volunteer to help out with booths, odd jobs, and cooking. Deb, already my friend, was in charge of cooking and asked if I would help in the fajita booth.

"Sure," I said.

I liked Deb and appreciated her wonderful organizational skills. So the day before Yesterfest I showed up to do whatever she wanted me to do. Kelly arrived at the same time I did, and she sent us off to pick up a cord of hardwood for the grill.

Kelly and I hopped in my pickup truck and off we went on a twenty-mile round trip to load and transport wood. He seemed like a nice young man, one of those loose-jointed youngsters who, though I didn't know it at the time, was to become a friend of mine. He looked about twenty years old, although he was more than ten years older.

But Kelly was nervous. Now I'm not really that scary, but if he could have pushed out the passenger door to put more room between us, I think he would have. To make matters worse, I started to ask him a zillion questions. Perhaps it seemed like the third degree, but I was curious about him, and he seemed willing to respond. I soon figured out that he surely was ADD. That took about three minutes and cost him nothing. (As already noted, ADD people are often attracted to other ADD people—like magnets; that's what happened between Kelly and me.) We ended up in a playful mood as we hit it off, liking one another quickly.

Loading a cord of wood also helps you get acquainted with a person. We worked easily together and by the time we'd unloaded the wood at the other end, I knew I wanted to give Kelly a helping hand to get his ADD in order. But I don't feel comfortable going up to people on the street and saying, "Oh, by the way, I think you're ADD. Want some help?"

Later that day, when Deb and I were standing together, I asked her, "Does Kelly know he's ADD?"

She responded in a matter-of-fact, blunt, loving, but this-is-all-business tone, "Not yet." I knew the matter was taken care of. That's the kind of confidence I have in Deb. And I knew she would do a good job helping Kelly begin to get what he needed.

Here's how she accomplished it. "I had your books at home," she said to me "and laid them out on the table. He picked up the one he wanted to."

Kelly adds at this point, "It's like how I'm trying to help a guy at work now. I want to tell him, 'You're ADD,' but I can't just come out and say it. Instead, I've said, 'Hey, you're just like me. You don't know how much you're like me.'

"I try to explain to him in situations where his ADD is getting in the way that I used to be that way, but so far, he's not hearing me."

However, Kelly did hear Deb. He was open and got the idea right away. And it wasn't long after Yesterfest that Kelly was formally evaluated for ADD. Kelly, my new friend, began to hang out at my place and we traded yard and repair work for guidance about handling his ADD. His relationship to Deb was growing and she, too, was able to help him get information about how to stabilize his life.

Because of their age difference, Deb and Kelly have an unusual situation. She doesn't mother him any more than I do as a friend. But she is an information giver, supporter, and all-around cheer-leader who doesn't take "nothing off of nobody." That's what experience has taught her.

As she says it, "I didn't really do anything for Kelly. He did things on his own that began to bring the chaos of his life under control. I was just behind him saying, 'Are you sure that's the way you want to go?'"

To this day, Deb and Kelly are hesitant to acknowledge the depth of their relationship. Laughingly, they say how scared they are of commitment. "We have a kind of 'anti-nuptial agreement,' which means we are both scared about getting tied into another marriage," says Deb.

"We're not really going together," affirms Kelly.

Most of the rest of us around them have seen the love, com-panionship, and friendship flourish, but Deb and Kelly insist,

"We aren't really a duo." Yeah, and birds don't fly! As I write this I can hear them laughing and looking shyly at each other. Trust is a hard nut to crack.

How Kelly and Deb Envision the Future

When thinking about the future, Kelly doesn't hesitate. "Fifty acres in the Rocky Mountains with some horses and cattle would suit me just fine," he says. That's his dream. It has been for some time and, I suspect, will be until he gets it. When I tell him this, he nods his head positively while a sweet light appears in his eyes.

When asked about plans for making a living, Kelly laughs. "Who said anything about making a living? In my dream, you've got firewood. You've got heating. You've got cattle. You can grow corn." Then a little more seriously, he adds, "I know I have to have an initial investment. That's what this city job is about."

Practical Deb pops in at this point. "What about the hay and the feed? You have to have running water and electricity." Then she adds, "What about a refrigerator to store your feed in? What about a car? Or are you going to ride your horse into town? Oh yeah, you gotta feed that horse, too. And you gotta have a barn."

Not to be deterred, Kelly quickly comes back with a broad grin on his face. "That's why I'm working now. I've got benefits, and I am building the life I want for the future. Now I know I can do it."

Deb smiles softly at his remark, communicating her pleasure at the progress he's made in the last year and a half.

Poetry, drawing and painting are again calling to Kelly in his off hours, of which there aren't many, but he'll sneak time when he can. Interested in these as a child, he has not pursued them since his teachers accused him of tracing the pictures he had drawn.

He's saving his money to buy art supplies and wants to learn woodcarving. Kelly's creative juices are just beginning to flow again, aided by the stability of getting his daily living under control.

Deb's future is tied to the job she's had for nearly a year and a half as a bail bondsperson. She's finally found her niche and likes the opportunities to work in a job where she can use her talents, brains, and experiences.

She's settled down a lot since being with Kelly and isn't looking for a lot of changes other than buying some land so that she can build her own home rather than being a renter. A good money manager, except when she loans money to people who may or may not pay it back, she can figure out what she needs and how long it will take her.

Kelly and Deb are planning to continue their relationship of love. But part of their future includes a joint decision for Kelly to "be more on his own." He is ready to take responsibility for his own place and is looking into making and keeping a budget, jobs that Deb has thus far performed. He's even playing with ideas for how he wants to decorate his own living area.

Kelly's daughter, still a preschooler, is another big part of both Kelly's and Deb's future. Kelly wants to be very active in her raising. Having his own place is important to him in part so that Kelsie can live with him full-time. An intuitively good, loving parent, Kelly knows what he wants to give her and is taking steps in that direction. And he and Deb are clear that Kelsie is Kelly's responsibility—not Deb's.

Only time will tell how Kelly and Deb's living relationship will work out. But as friends and soul mates they are committed indefinitely.

What's really nice is to see how honest and out front they are with each other as they face their individual futures and honor one another. True love and caring for each other shines between Kelly and Deb, so much so that they can let go of each other if that should prove to be in the best interest of either. Meanwhile, they'll continue to walk parallel paths, mutually supporting and loving one another.

What Works For and Against Kelly

Which of his ADD traits is the most positive in Kelly's life? "His playfulness," Deb volunteers immediately. "That's what attracted me to him in the first place. Of course, I'm sure there was something much more physical going on, too. But he was a special pleasure to be around. He was and still is very childlike. I like that."

Next Deb talks about what Kelly provides for her emotionally. "He gives me the opportunity to reexperience something that I had once known but had forgotten. It's the wonderment," she says. "The discovery. I was very hurt in my last marriage. It was tough. I was pretty gun-shy.

"Kelly's the classic protector. Almost to the point of smothering me at times—he wants to make sure that I get the best of everything even if I don't know it's the best. He may make judgment calls for me even though he may not know what's best. Like when I get very involved with one of my bail bond clients, and he sees I'm likely to get hurt. He reminds me to back off. I understand why he does this, to protect me."

She continues, not needing any prompting, "Last winter when it was icy, he insisted on backing my car out of our driveway. Or, at least, he tried. He couldn't get it out either because of the ice, but he felt better having tried. Even though I knew neither of us was going to get out that morning, it was sweet to see him give it a try. He's very persistent as well as protective."

Kelly's intuition and sensitivity are finding places to be used as his network of friends, acquaintances, and co-workers becomes more extensive. By getting his temper under control, he attracts people who are also sensitive and as a result is learning to channel his people skills.

Though he's always had ADD sensitivity and people-awareness, he's just now learning to use them constructively. Previously, no one had taught him how to handle them. He simply didn't have the language or concepts of what to do with all those feelings he felt inside himself. Deb to a large extent has been responsible for providing him with a vocabulary that helps him now.

Kelly's biggest drawback has been his temper. Previously it went unchecked. Now thanks to anger management classes, a new vocabulary, and time to practice ADD temper-control steps, he can keep himself from getting into big trouble with it.

Smiling, Kelly says, "My sensitivity. The guys at work play with everybody. They have their ways of doing things. To me they'll say something that really hurts my feelings. But because of the circumstances that I'm in, I can't really show it. I gotta play it off as a joke, and go along with them, or I lose my temper.

"Let me give you an example. The other day I was sitting in the break room. Everyone was there eating lunch. This one guy who technically is supposed to be over me, but I've been told not to listen to him, opened the refrigerator door. I didn't look at him, but I could feel what he was doing. Next he opened up the freezer and there was his butt just an inch away from my face and he let go, right there. Yeah! He farted, right in my face.

"The guy said, 'Gee, I'm sorry.' I come up out of the chair and come unglued on him. I said, 'Don't even play these childish games with me anymore. I'm not . . .'

"I was so mad that when I stood up out of that chair everybody in the room thought I was going to whoop his ass, right there. The expression in my face. My boss was grabbing his food, because he was going to move."

Hearing this, I ask Kelly, "What kept you from whipping his butt?"

He responds after a long hesitation. "That's a hard question."

With tears in my eyes, I say, "That's how far you've come."

"What do you mean?" Kelly asks.

"That's how far you've come in your quest to gain control over your life."

As Kelly begins to understand what I am talking about, his eyebrows rise. He looks up innocently with amazement and says, "Oh, yeah. My anger especially. I mean, I don't know why. It just . . . wasn't proper to do it just then."

"You know, Kelly," I say, "That doesn't mean that you don't get angry because someone farts in your face. That's real normal. The fact is you had control, and my tears are because if you had come unglued, even though you were justified, you could still have gotten in trouble."

At that point Kelly adds, "I'd probably have lost my job."

So even though Kelly still has a temper, he is managing to keep it under control. And he has the ability to talk out his feelings with friends.

Other than his temper, which he is managing, Kelly's obstacles come more from inexperience than from bad habits. "He's learning the ways of the world, politics and stuff like that," says Deb. She gives an example of a discussion they'd had recently. It seems that Kelly's boss had said, "You know the city manager has been watching you out his window and has been very impressed with all those busy bees down by the river."

She continues to relate, "Kelly was excited because he's really trying to do a super job and the thought that he was being recognized pleased him." Then she tells how she had to point out to Kelly what was really going on. She told him, "The city manager's office is on the other side of the building, and there are no windows." To that she says, "Kelly looked puzzled."

Explaining further, Deb played the role that she often plays with him, saying, "Kelly, this is the third time that your boss has started to razz you and that means that someone is coming to check on your work—politics. Your boss says it in a teasing way, but what he's really telling you is 'Be prepared.'"

With this introduction to politics on the job and the subtleties of people's communications, Kelly has begun to listen differently to what people say. Though deciphering those kinds of messages is not natural to someone with ADD wiring, Kelly is learning how to do it. He realizes that, like it or not, if he wants to reach his goals, he must learn the secondary language of the job. And he's willing.

WHAT KELLY AND DEB WANT YOU TO KNOW

FROM KELLY

Get information about ADD.

Forget that deficit stuff.

Be creative.

Open yourself to more of nature and the way nature is.

Use humor.

FROM DEB

Make it safe for tenderness.

Learn nonverbal communication.

Love.

Respect.

Use humor.

Be prepared to change.

B.J. and Ken Pailer

I didn't used to know what was important to me. Now I know. BJP

She didn't know how to manage money. KP

Now her work provides her with a paycheck of the heart, so both she and Ken are happy. LW

ADD affects people throughout their life span. It affects their children and their children's children. Sometimes the effects are not pretty. Sometimes, those who have been blessed with early support and direction don't understand what it's like to be lost— lost all your life—trying simply to survive without knowing how to do that or what to do to make things better.

The couple in this story are willing to tell their story so that others may learn how hard it can be. This is not as pretty a story as some in this book. It may even offend you if you believe people can always have control over their thoughts and actions, not realizing that this control is learned.

B.J., a fifty-five-year-old Florida woman, functioned pretty well as a child but got into trouble when she entered the unstructured world of adulthood at age eighteen. Faced with too many choices and no mentors or guidelines to help her, she began a downward spiral that took over thirty-five years to pull out of. Ken, B.J.'s second husband, now in his early seventies, didn't understand much about feelings or sensitive, intimate relations with someone you love. He didn't realize what his wife needed in order to live successfully. And neither of them knew how to communicate or what to do to make things better.

It's not popular for a mother to have such overwhelming emotional needs that she doesn't pay attention to her children's needs. Yet it is much more common than many people realize. It's looked down upon to have affairs, but people do it all the time. It's not acceptable to drink too much, lie, or spend money uncontrollably. And if you do have any of these behaviors, it's certainly not nice to talk about them.

The difference between B.J. and Ken and many other couples is that they are willing to tell the truth about a background that "looks bad," rather than hide behind a mask of silence, pretending that all is well and always has been. Until B.J.'s ADD was identified in 1994, neither she nor Ken would have been considered as candidates for this book. But the work each has done since then establishes them in my mind as an appropriate choice to speak to the many readers who may need hope because their own lives are in such chaos. Inspiration is my main goal in sharing B.J.'s and Ken's story. If they can make it, so can anyone else.

But perhaps most heartwarming is the effect their recovery has had on their family. Their children, now adults with their own histories of drug and alcohol abuse, poor relationships, and less than exemplary behavior, have begun to recover their health and lost potential—in large part because of the healing work B.J. and Ken initiated. The intergenerational effects of unrecognized, unguided ADD are coming to an end in this family. It can be stopped whenever someone knows to stop it, knows what to do and how to do it.

"When I'm desperate, I do stupid things." The words caught my attention big time. The tone of B.J.'s voice was somber, and I knew there had to be a very big, probably sad, story behind her matter-of-fact remark. And indeed there is.

B.J.'s dark hair frames the face of a vibrant woman who's a great talker and skillful teacher. B.J. conveys the image of a woman who has many talents and has accomplished a lot. Add to that the fact that she is extremely bright as well as creative, and it's hard to believe that she hasn't always lived a happy, constructive life.

But the truth is that only three years ago, she was chewing on ice prior to being wheeled into the operating room for major surgery. As a registered nurse, she knew that the surgery would be canceled if she didn't bring down the temperature she was running. So she ate the ice to disguise the temperature. It wasn't that she was that eager to have the surgery. Rather, she wanted to die. She figured that if she had a temperature prior to the operation, she'd run a better chance of not surviving.

Convoluted thinking? Maybe. But what she and I both realize now is how much emotional pain she was in at the time. She wasn't crazy, just suffering major grief over the loss of a creative business and guilt about having "run away," letting her children down during their teen years. She also became afraid of facing a growing feeling of hatred for her husband, Ken.

In combination, these pressures proved too much for her, and she just wanted to die—the ultimate runaway.

Well, B.J. didn't die. In fact she woke up to find a Catholic priest sitting by her bedside and realized that since she was still alive, she'd better begin to find out what was wrong—why did she feel so bad? That's what the last three years have been about.

B.J.'s Background

"I grew up everywhere," reflects B.J., displaying her wonderfully expansive mind. It is also nearly true. Attending eight different schools in third grade alone certainly supports the perception that she lived everywhere.

You might guess that B.J.'s father was in the military. B.J.'s mother was completely deaf and followed her husband around to remote areas of the world. B.J. and her sister, four years younger, had few roots and little consistent day-to-day opportunity to learn what it felt like to count on much of anything. In between assignments, B.J., her sister, and their mother would go back to their mother's family until they'd be thrown out. Then they'd move on again. With little structure to her schooling, B.J. did a lot of self-learning. One school experience does stands out in her mind, though. Sporadically she lived with her father's family in Birmingham, Alabama, and went to a one-room school house. She says, "I spent most of my second grade there and off and on other times. I loved the farm on the very top of the mountain overlooking the city. I knew everybody in school, could learn at my own pace and had freedom on the farm."

B.J. dearly needed the stability she briefly achieved in that old-fashioned school. Consistently contained in one room, guided gently, she knew what to do and felt secure. Otherwise it was move, move, move. B.J.'s family finally relocated to Pensacola, Florida, when she was in the seventh grade. She stayed there until she graduated from high school.

Peace and stability were short-lived for B.J., however. During her last year in high school, her father insisted that she go to secretarial school so that she could be assured of a good job. "I was always strongly influenced by him so I did it," says B.J. "But I also wanted to go to college so I finished regular high school at the same time."

Her senior year in high school was a major turning point in her life. Besides completing the two school programs, she worked in a law office and went steady with the boyfriend she'd dated from the time she was fourteen. She thought they would marry.

Then, on top of all that, she was offered a full college scholarship. But B.J. was unable to make a decision to do what she really wanted. Faced with too many options, she experienced what many young ADD people go through—a feeling of being totally overwhelmed. It's called flooding.

B.J. took the easiest path out of the confusion that she could find. She stayed in the job she already had rather than risking doing anything new. After all, she expected to be married soon. But weeks before the marriage date, with invitations already mailed, the boyfriend called to tell her he had married someone else. It was at that point that B.J. "did something stupid" out of desperation. She went out with a school chum who'd just broken up with his girlfriend; she got drunk and pregnant. As she tells it, "It was just one night. We never dated before or after, but my mother made sure we got married. It lasted three weeks. We moved to another part of Florida where he walked out on me when I was five months pregnant. He took all of my money, so I went home again."

B.J. spent the next couple of years feeling confused and desperate. Unfortunately, she tended to act out her feelings, an ADD tendency when a person has not been helped to learn to manage feelings in other ways.

Her impulsive behavior led B.J. into a marriage of convenience—one that was less than perfect—by the age of twenty-two. With three children by then, B.J. says, "We were starving to death, so I went out to get a job."

It was then that she met Ken Pailer. She instantly fell in love with his blue eyes and went to work for him. Completely acting on her feelings, B.J. says, "I'd never really loved anyone like that. This was soul mate time." However, both she and Ken were already married. Neither could resist the feelings, and they started an affair that lasted over two years. It only ended when Ken retired from the military and moved.

Ken Pailer, the oldest of three children, grew up in Baltimore, Maryland. His life was totally different from B.J.'s. His family and life were stable. Ken went to the high school of his choice, determined to follow his passion of becoming an airline pilot. He says,

"I wanted to do that after being taken to the local airport when I was seven years old. From then on I built model airplanes and became a Junior Birdman, signing up for a correspondence class that gave flight lessons to children. With this highly focused dream, he went into the navy in World War II to become a pilot. He flew for twenty-five years for the navy before retiring from the service. He continued to fly for another fifteen years as a civilian.

But Ken was a novice when it came to feelings and sensitive interpersonal relations. Engineering, tactical planning, and incredible attention to detail did not leave room for the intricacies and subtleties of becoming aware of how feelings work or the fact that love and passion can be expressed in many different ways.

Ken did marry right after World War II, "because it was the thing to do." Thirty-one years of marriage ended with his wife's death. He and his wife had one daughter.

After Ken's retirement and move, B.J., still married, decided to return to school. About that time, her eight-year-old son was diagnosed with minimal brain dysfunction (as earlier noted, this was an old term for ADD). Her son's doctor realized that B.J. was interested in learning all she could about her son's problems. He was impressed with her inquisitiveness and arranged for B.J. to receive a scholarship to nursing school.

Although she wasn't particularly drawn to nursing, she decided to go ahead because it was a practical route to take. Again, she did not follow her heart, but followed what an authority figure suggested.

About that time, B.J. decided to divorce her husband, move across town closer to school, and begin her college studies. After six months, she and her ex-husband reconciled. No sooner was that accomplished than he was diagnosed with cancer, which meant that her two years of nursing school included home care for her husband. He died three years after being diagnosed.

Despite all this, nursing school remained a top priority. "I was just reacting, though, not planning. Now I see that I 'settled,' which is what a lot of ADD people do. I avoided taking responsibility for my life. I didn't know how." But, I must add, B.J. survived and honored her priority.

The year before her husband died, B.J. had graduated and was working alternate day and night shifts. They had no money. "The day of the funeral, I had to use a credit card to eat breakfast with the kids.

"I wasn't able to face nursing, but creditors were everywhere after my husband's lengthy illness. My solution was to go back to doing secretarial work. I had no support from my family, and I got heavy into alcohol, heavy into withdrawal, became real promiscuous, and headed back to my old boy friends, including my first ex-husband. It was then that Ken showed up."

Flying for a commuter airline after retirement, Ken hadn't seen B.J. for ten years. It was at his wife's funeral that someone told him B.J. was living nearby. He waited a couple of weeks and went to try and find her.

Ken says, "I drove around to where I thought her place was. When I couldn't find it, I stopped a little tow-headed boy on the street and asked if he knew where she lived. The child said, 'I'll show you where it is.'" The boy turned out to be B.J.'s youngest son, and he took Ken right to her door. They agreed to see each other on her birthday two weeks later. They've been together ever since. But it's not been all smooth sailing.

It was three years before they got married. Ken didn't get along with B.J.'s kids, who were in their teens by then. Her oldest son was on cocaine. There were a lot of family problems. B.J. still wasn't working at anything that she loved. She'd never gotten stabilized after her husband's death.

"With Ken I was trying to live two lives," says B.J. "I kept trying to keep him and the kids apart. I was trying to be a girlfriend to Ken and a mother to the kids, who were sixteen, fourteen, and thirteen. The kids got put on the back burner while

Ken and I partied a lot"—a fact that has bothered B.J. for many years.

But she wasn't able to do anything to right the situation until after she was diagnosed with ADD. Only then, twenty-five years later and thanks to training, education, and medication, did she become able to think clearly enough to handle more than one thing at a time. Only then was she able to develop the maturity that could put her children's needs before her own.

At the time, B.J. was trying to figure out what to do but couldn't think straight enough to do anything but run away. She says, "Ken and I got on a sailboat and ran away and left everyone. I still feel guilty about abandoning my sons. It was the biggest mistake I've ever made in my life."

Ken, less tuned in to the psychological implications of their leaving, thinks he and B.J. did handle the pragmatics of the situation. "We didn't exactly leave those kids. We asked them to move with us but they refused. They stayed in Pensacola while we went to Key Largo. Because I flew for an air cargo company, we got passes so B.J. could be back in Pensacola in an hour and a half. We sent them money. And they were living in a big house and later a townhouse. We took care of them. The two younger sons went to college."

But B.J. retorts, "The bad part was I missed their junior and senior years in high school." Now B.J. realizes that the boys needed her emotionally and she needed to be with them. They didn't just need "things" but the presence of a parent or parents who cared. At the time, she probably knew these things intuitively, which is why she felt guilty, but she couldn't do anything about meeting their needs.

Ken, on the other hand, didn't realize the difference between giving things and supplying firsthand personal care. He knows now.

"I did love being on the yacht. I felt better there. But the guilt about the kids ate at me," B.J. says. "I started a long process of learning to hate Ken. I was too torn between him and the boys. Now I realize that I can't blame Ken for making me go with him. I did leave him a few times but would be back within hours. I just couldn't break away. I allowed it to happen. I could have said no. I should have said, 'I have to stay here. I have obligations as a mother.'"

B.J. and Ken returned to land in 1987 after five years living on their yacht. An adrenal gland problem caused heart complications that required medical attention for B.J. They moved back to Pensacola. Once her health was stabilized, B.J. tried nursing again. But after three years, she found that she was still unhappy with it and decided to exercise her creative talents. She started to design women's clothing.

According to both of them, her fashions were "beautiful," but B.J. could neither manage the marketing nor handle the money aspects of the business. Because she and Ken had not yet learned to communicate their feelings or ask each other for help, they looked at the business differently. And B.J. got herself into big financial trouble.

Ken felt frustrated as he watched money going rapidly down the drain. B.J. felt that Ken was unfairly trying to control her. Their situation came to a head when Ken received a call from the bank. The caller apologized for not being able to extend Ken's credit limit on his card, and Ken replied, "I don't have a card with your bank." The man said, "Oh yes, you do."

It turns out that B.J., by her own admission, had forged Ken's signature and run up the card. This is how she explains it. "It seems I started out with two credit cards. Pretty soon, these were maxed out, and I had no money to make the payments, so I had to get another card to make the payments."

Six months and $26,000 later, Ken got the wake-up call. He didn't laugh then. He laughs now. "She never missed a payment, which was good in one respect." Their credit remained excellent. "He agreed to pay off the cards if I would cut them up," says B.J.

Feeling disgraced, guilty, and a failure she wanted to "check out"; she hoped to end her life by dying on the operating table early in 1994. But when B.J. didn't die, she became determined to turn her life around.

That year became a busy year of change. She left Ken. It was an amicable separation that was to last a year. She began taking classes at the spouse abuse program but soon discovered that there was a big difference between being a battered woman and being the recipient of verbal abuse that she perceived was coming from Ken. Ken attended anger management classes for six sessions and began to get some insight into his feelings. He says, "I discovered I wasn't angry, but I also began to realize that B.J. and I had major communication problems."

As B.J. continued to seek her answers about what was wrong with her and Ken, she came to a realization. "It is true that he was often thoughtless and unaware, but he wasn't abusive. He didn't realize how emotionally distressed I was. He had to learn, and has learned to read me well.

"I had already begun to change how I looked at our situation when the possibility surfaced in September of 1994 of unidentified, untreated ADD being a contributor to my problems."

Ken notes, "By late October of 1994, I received a call from B.J. to join her for a discussion. We decided to have a temporary reconciliation on a trial basis to see what would happen. We both received counseling after that, and B.J. started medication to help her get her ADD under control."

Their relationship finally began to improve and became better than ever. They were remarried in the Catholic church and were united emotionally on a level neither had known before. They became a team.

Today they are a very happy, healthy couple who have learned to respect each other and to take responsibility for their own actions.

The difficulties between Ken and B.J.'s children have resolved themselves, but it has taken time. B.J. says, "Ken has become more tolerant, since knowing about my son's ADD. He's not taking the young man's behavior personally." She, in turn, has been able to pass on to her son what she has learned and together they are learning to manage their lives.

B.J. smiles, as she talks about her youngest son, the tow-headed kid who led Ken to her house many years before. It seems he is emulating Ken: he's become a navy pilot and spends more time talking to Ken than to B.J. these days. They have a lot in common. So, Ken, the man who never much cared about children, is getting a new perspective on adult children.

B.J. loves sharing how she and Ken now handle ADD problems that used to create hassles between them. "Now, for example," she says, he and I both have skills and cues we use with each other that allow us to communicate even when we are under stress. For example, if I get talking too much at the club, Ken has my permission to bump me on the knee to let me know. That's an example of our deals. I never knew such skills existed, much less learned them."

B.J. proudly says, "I no longer lie to Ken. I'm more trusting and very much more honest. I am now aware of my value system. I never knew about having one before. I know now that I need acknowledgment for what I can do. I need that a lot and never got it before. I kept doing things to try to get it, but never knew how to get it the right way.

"I understand now that number one on Ken's list is money because of the depression and all that he's lived through. Though he never went hungry as a child, often his father had to work three jobs and money was tight. He also understands about money and can keep track of it. I never could.

"Before, anything having to do with money would put us at odds. Now I respect the fact that it is ingrained in his soul, and I owe him the respect to let him know what's happening with the money. And since we're working together, finally, he helps me keep track of it. I can count on him.

"I do take medication. That helps, especially at the beginning, so I could focus more and settle down to learn the new skills I needed to know. But it's having the knowledge and knowing the tools to manage my ADD attributes that's also made me able to change. For example, knowing how to keep from interrupting people has made a big difference."

Ken notices differences, too. "It's how she functions. She's so much better to live with. She doesn't take the wrong meaning out of things I say. The whole thing [living together] seems more relaxing. I'm not walking on eggs all the time any more."

They now teach the skills they've learned in B.J.'s ADD skill-building classes. Working together has led to their truly respecting each other's talents. Ken says, "I like to watch people's faces and see them responding to B.J. We talk about it afterwards. I'm kind of a confidentiality partner for her."

At that B.J. chimes in and brags on Ken. "Not only does he take the money and make sure everybody pays when they come to class, but he sets up the classroom, does the banking, and sees everybody leaves the meeting on time. But more importantly, he takes the spouses and partners of ADD people aside and helps them—he talks with them, sometimes for hours. He really helps. We're a team now."

B.J. and Ken are like a couple of kids learning new skills. In many ways that's exactly what's happening. B.J. is getting the direction and limits she never knew. Ken is coming to understand about feelings and emotional depth. Both have found something they love to do and do well together.

It's fun to be around them and listen to each bragging about the other. They are able to share the love they first felt for one another, but now they have the skills to live together so that love can blossom rather than wither. It's no longer an exclusive love that pushes their family members away. It's an expansive love that has actually pulled their children into the fold, healing two generations.

Just last Christmas, the whole family came together: her three sons and her sister; his daughter and her mother. B.J. says, "For the first time, everyone is healthy emotionally. No one is using drugs or alcohol. Everyone has become responsible and we all get along great.

"We understand what it used to be like and we like this a lot better. There was a lot of forgiveness going on for past mistakes and a lot of learning to handle current situations. We are all sharing what we know and helping one another. It sure feels good."

How I First Met B.J. and Ken

There I was at a national ADD conference wandering around at a "meet and greet" reception. An affable couple approached me with such outgoing exuberance that I thought I'd probably met them before—I just couldn't remember where or when. Actually I hadn't, but I now realize that's how gregarious they are.

B.J. was wide-eyed, talkative, and very enthusiastic about ADD. Bright, very hyperactive, and a terrific networker, eight months after her diagnosis she'd already begun to make ADD her business, first for herself and later so that she could help others. Ken was quieter as we sat and talked, but he seemed interested, had a good sense of humor, and appeared affirming of his wife.

B. J. wanted to have me come to Pensacola to conduct a public meeting and provide in-service training with the private non-profit center where she'd been teaching ADD classes. A true believer in what training and education can do to change the way people feel and act, B.J. was on a mission to spread the word about ADD. Considering her own painful past, is it any wonder?

What I didn't know at the time was how much B.J. had changed. I had no idea of the chaos that had been present most of her life. Instead I found a well-organized B.J. who brought her plan to fruition within the year. I also discovered a supportive, caring husband who has made it his business to learn as much as he could about ADD. He took on the assignment of doing all the detail work to make his wife's projects succeed. Little did I know how much he, too, had changed.

Since then, B.J. has built her business by networking with agencies and businesses in her community. She's sponsored training groups for professionals in the community, run groups for people identified with ADD, and become an ADD coach. She and Ken have continued to join forces and, often working as a team, provide a model for couples who want to make their marriages and personal lives better. There isn't much they haven't experienced firsthand themselves. That makes them helpful and optimistic even when confronted with the darkest-appearing situations. Having seen the light at the end of their own tunnel, they are able to see the light in others. This is their gift.

How B.J. and Ken Envision the Future

Ken jumps right in saying, "I see B.J. continuing with her latest enterprise, her ADD business. For me, I'd like enough time in the future to get a bass boat and take a little time off."

On the heels of his comment, B.J. interjects, "He'd like me to be successful money-wise."

Sympathetically, Ken drawls, "Well, yes." Then caringly, he adds, "A couple of times she's gotten a little discouraged. I don't think she really meant it, but she wanted to shut her ADD business down." Then, emphatically, he says, "I'm not going to let her, because she does so well at it."

So with that support, I ask B.J. what discourages her. "Being overwhelmed" is her response. "I'm the only person doing the ADD skill-building training and networking here. And a few months ago Ken became ill. That drained me some. But he's better now."

She continues, "People I'd been helping sometimes let me down. That discourages me. It sets me back a little, though not like it used to. Now I'm more determined than ever." B.J. plans to continue to educate the public and professionals about ADD and to train people in running skill-building groups.

What Works For and Against B.J.

Both B.J. and Ken mention her creativity as her major ADD attribute. She's both artistically creative and a talented program developer. She is a visionary who sees the big picture while envisioning how to connect with the status quo. Only now she can make use of her creativity effectively.

Humor and high energy stand B.J. in good stead. Verbally, she is a dynamo. Physically, she romps around like someone half her age. Every once in a while, Ken gently guides her toward self-care and rest, which she now accepts graciously. He doesn't mind playing a protective role—actually he rather likes it, as he sequesters her away from the many demands on her time and energy.

Through teamwork, she no longer gets herself overwhelmed to the degree she once did. Both she and Ken know better than to let that happen. And they now know what to do to stop it from escalating.

B.J. appreciates her ADD traits of friendliness, sociability, and outgoingness. She uses them regularly to do the work she has come to love. She says, "I also use the lack of boundaries that are so common with ADD people to help me pick up a phone and call people I don't know, even people who may be well-known. It doesn't matter to me that I don't know them at all. I call anyway. And I get terrific responses."

And these same people seem to recognize that her intent is good, her heart is big, and she is someone who can be trusted. They do respond.

B.J.'s sensitivity contributes greatly to her success. "I am sensitive to what a situation needs, to what another person needs and to what the world needs," B.J. says. "It's the crux of why I'm very successful working in the ADD business."

I might add, she now knows what she needs too. B.J. has managed to turn her early sensitivity around into a positive attribute so that she no longer gets into trouble because of it. Amazing as it may seem, much of her early difficulty stemmed from being too sensitive without having any idea what to do to protect herself. So she became overwhelmed and went off in all directions.

Ken immediately jumps on the bandwagon. "She sure reads me very well. Without having to tell her, she reads my mind. I can't get away with anything." At that he laughs a hearty laugh, a Ken laugh, and we all chuckle.

Even B.J.'s impulsivity, which used to be so much of a problem, is really quite under control now. And Ken has been a part of that change, too. B.J. says, "I don't do anything major any more, anything that involves hundreds of dollars, without talking to Ken first. It's not that he makes me. I use him to think through my purchases."

When I ask Ken what B.J. still has to work on, he says, "Interrupting." With a sound of affection in his voice, he adds, "She'll get to talking too much if her Ritalin has worn off. That's when I have permission to bump her on the knee or ring a bell or something."

So, in reality, B.J. and Ken have managed to get her ADD attributes under control, using them for constructive purposes in most instances. And when an unconstructive trait slips through, they work together to curb it so that it does not cause trouble.

Ken, in turn, has learned a lot more about feelings because of his sensitive ADD wife. And as a result, their whole family has benefited, as have the people with whom they work professionally. Good teamwork!

WHAT B.J. AND KEN WANT YOU TO KNOW

From B.J.

Be honest.

Talk out your differences.

Focus on what to do about your ADD not on the diagnosis.
Don't get hung up on medication as a magic pill.

Get training.

Embrace your ADD.

From Ken

Find out as much as you can about ADD.

Don't use ADD as a hammer or an excuse.

Admire the creativity of ADD.